# Handbook of obstetric high dependency care

**David Vaughan**
**Neville Robinson**
**Nuala Lucas**
**Sabaratnam Arulkumaran**

WILEY-BLACKWELL

A John Wiley & Sons, Ltd., Publication

This edition first published 2010, © 2010 by David Vaughan, Neville Robinson, Nuala Lucas, Sabaratnam Arulkumaran

Blackwell Publishing was acquired by John Wiley & Sons in February 2007. Blackwell's publishing program has been merged with Wiley's global Scientific, Technical and Medical business to form Wiley-Blackwell.

Registered office: John Wiley & Sons Ltd, The Atrium, Southern Gate, Chichester, West Sussex, PO19 8SQ, UK

Editorial offices: 9600 Garsington Road, Oxford, OX4 2DQ, UK
111 River Street, Hoboken, NJ 07030-5774, USA
The Atrium, Southern Gate, Chichester, West Sussex, PO19 8SQ, UK

For details of our global editorial offices, for customer services and for information about how to apply for permission to reuse the copyright material in this book please see our website at www.wiley.com/wiley-blackwell

The right of the author to be identified as the author of this work has been asserted in accordance with the Copyright, Designs and Patents Act 1988.

Wiley also publishes its books in a variety of electronic formats. Some content that appears in print may not be available in electronic books.

Designations used by companies to distinguish their products are often claimed as trademarks. All brand names and product names used in this book are trade names, service marks, trademarks or registered trademarks of their respective owners. The publisher is not associated with any product or vendor mentioned in this book. This publication is designed to provide accurate and authoritative information in regard to the subject matter covered. It is sold on the understanding that the publisher is not engaged in rendering professional services. If professional advice or other expert assistance is required, the services of a competent professional should be sought.

The contents of this work are intended to further general scientific research, understanding, and discussion only and are not intended and should not be relied upon as recommending or promoting a specific method, diagnosis, or treatment by physicians for any particular patient. The publisher and the author make no representations or warranties with respect to the accuracy or completeness of the contents of this work and specifically disclaim all warranties, including without limitation any implied warranties of fitness for a particular purpose. In view of ongoing research, equipment modifications, changes in governmental regulations, and the constant flow of information relating to the use of medicines, equipment, and devices, the reader is urged to review and evaluate the information provided in the package insert or instructions for each medicine, equipment, or device for, among other things, any changes in the instructions or indication of usage and for added warnings and precautions. Readers should consult with a specialist where appropriate. The fact that an organization or Website is referred to in this work as a citation and/or a potential source of further information does not mean that the author or the publisher endorses the information the organization or Website may provide or recommendations it may make. Further, readers should be aware that Internet Websites listed in this work may have changed or disappeared between when this work was written and when it is read. No warranty may be created or extended by any promotional statements for this work. Neither the publisher nor the author shall be liable for any damages arising herefrom.

Library of Congress Cataloging-in-Publication Data

Handbook of obstetric high dependency care / David Vaughan ... [et al.].
p. ; cm.
Includes bibliographical references and index.
ISBN 978-1-4051-7821-1 (pbk.)
1. Pregnancy—Complications—Handbooks, manuals, etc. 2. Obstetrics—Handbooks, manuals, etc. 3. Critical care medicine—Handbooks, manuals, etc. I. Vaughan, David, MBBS.
[DNLM: 1. Pregnancy Complications—therapy. 2. Critical Care—methods. WQ 240 H2365 2010]
RG573.H36 2010
618.2—dc22

2010023981

ISBN: 978-1-4051-7821-1

A catalogue record for this book is available from the British Library.

Set in 9.25/12pt Meridien by MPS Limited, A Macmillan Company

Printed and bound in Singapore by Fabulous Printers Pte Ltd

1  2010

# Contents

# List of abbreviations

We have endeavoured to expand all abbreviations used in the text, but for ease of reference the more common are listed below.

| | |
|---|---|
| AAGBI | Association of Anaesthetists of Great Britain and Ireland |
| ABC/ABCDE | Steps of emergency assessment/resuscitation – airway, breathing, circulation, disability, exposure |
| ACE | angiotensin-converting enzyme |
| AF | atrial fibrillation |
| AFLP | acute fatty liver of pregnancy |
| ALS | advanced life support |
| ALT | alanine transaminase |
| AP | anteroposterior |
| APGAR | quick vital sign scoring system for newborn babies |
| ARF | acute renal failure |
| AST | aspartate transaminase |
| ATN | acute tubular necrosis |
| AVM | arteriovenous malformation |
| AVPU | CNS function quick assessment tool – Alert, responds to Verbal command, responds to Painful stimulus only, Unresponsive |
| BD | (latin – *bis die*) twice daily |
| BM | bedside blood sugar assay |
| BMI | body mass index ($kg/m^2$) |
| BP | blood pressure (mmHg) |
| Ca | calcium |
| CCrISP | care of the critically ill surgical patient |
| CMACE | Centre for Maternal and Child Enquiries |
| CEMACH | Confidential Enquiry into Maternal and Child Health |
| Cl | chlorine |
| cm $H_2O$ | pressure measurement |
| CNS | central nervous system |
| CNST | Clinical Negligence Scheme for Trusts |

| | |
|---|---|
| $CO_2$ | carbon dioxide |
| CPAP | continuous positive airway pressure |
| CPR | cardiopulmonary resuscitation |
| CRP | complement reactive protein serum assay |
| CSE | combined spinal-epidural |
| CT | computerised tomographic scan |
| CTG | cardiotocogram |
| CVS | cardiovascular system |
| CVP | central venous pressure |
| CXR | chest radiograph |
| DBP | diastolic blood pressure |
| DIC | disseminated intravascular coagulopathy |
| DVT | deep vein thrombosis |
| ECG | electrocardiogram |
| ENT | ear, nose and throat |
| FBC | full blood count |
| FFP | fresh frozen plasma |
| $FiO_2$ | fractional inspired oxygen (0.21 = air; 1.0 = 100% oxygen) |
| GCS | Glasgow coma score |
| GU | genitourinary |
| HBV | Hepatitis B virus |
| $HCO_3$ | bicarbonate |
| HDU | high dependency unit |
| HELLP | complication of pre-eclampsia; syndrome of haemolysis, elevated liver enzymes and low platelets |
| HIV | human immunodeficiency virus |
| HR | heart rate |
| ICU/ITU | intensive care/treatment unit |
| ID | internal diameter (usually related to endotracheal tube size in millimetres) |
| IM | intramuscular |
| IUGR | intrauterine growth restriction |
| IV | intravenous |
| K | potassium |
| LFT | serum assay of liver enzyme levels |
| LMWH | low molecular weight heparin |
| LSCS | lower segment caesarean section |
| MAP | mean arterial pressure |
| MEWS | maternal early warning score |
| MHDU | maternity high dependency unit |

| | |
|---|---|
| mmHg | millimetres of mercury – unit of pressure |
| MRI | magnetic resonance imaging |
| Na | sodium |
| NICE | National Institute for Clinical Excellence |
| NPSA | National Patient Safety Agency |
| NSAID | non-steroidal anti-inflammatory drug |
| $O_2$ | oxygen |
| OAA | Obstetric Anaesthetists Association |
| OD | (latin – *omni die*) once daily |
| P | pulse |
| PA | posteroanterior |
| $PaCO_2$ | partial pressure of arterial carbon dioxide |
| $PaO_2$ | partial pressure of arterial oxygen |
| PACS | picture archiving and communication system |
| PCA | patient-controlled analgesia |
| PE | pulmonary embolus |
| PET | pre-eclamptic toxaemia |
| pH | measure of blood acidity |
| PR | *either* (latin – *per rectum*) rectal examination or drug administration *or* relating to the 12-lead ECG the time between atrial and ventricular depolarisation |
| QDS | (latin – *quater die sumendus*) four times daily |
| QRS | part of the ECG representing ventricular depolarisation |
| RCA | Royal College of Anaesthetists |
| RCM | Royal College of Midwifery |
| RCOG | Royal College of Obstetricians and Gynaecologists |
| RCS | Royal College of Surgeons |
| RS | respiratory system |
| SAMM | severe acute maternal morbidity |
| $SaO_2$ | oxygen saturation (%) |
| SBP | systolic blood pressure |
| SIRS | systemic inflammatory response syndrome |
| SLE | systemic lupus erythematosis |
| ST | segment of ECG representing period of ventricular contraction |
| SVT | supraventricular tachycardia |
| TDS | (latin – *ter die sumendus*) three times daily |
| TED | thromboembolic disease – usually used to refer to preventative calf compression stockings |
| U&Es | renal blood profile – plasma urea, electrolyte and creatinine levels |

| VAS | visual analogue score |
| VF | ventricular fibrillation |
| V/Q | scan comparing lung ventilation and perfusion looking for areas of mismatch |
| VT | ventricular tachycardia |
| VTE | venous thromboembolism |
| WHO | World Health Organization |
| WPW | Wolff–Parkinson–White syndrome |

# List of figures

# List of boxes

# Preface

High dependency facilities are now an essential component of modern obstetric practice. The acutely ill parturient is now cared for by a multidisciplinary team within this specialised area. A patient does not present with a diagnosis but with an array of signs and symptoms which the staff caring for her must be able to detect, investigate and act upon.

This handbook aims to assist obstetricians, midwives, nurses and anaesthetists involved with the maternity high dependency unit in three ways: to provide an understanding of why these units are now a necessity to enhance safe obstetric care; to help obstetric units develop their own high dependency unit; and most importantly to assist with the treatment of clinical problems that occur in the ill parturient. It is not intended to be an exhaustive tome on the minutiae of obstetric pathology and medicine. However, we hope it will act as a practical bedside guide to help to achieve our goal of safer maternal care.

David Vaughan
Neville Robinson
Nuala Lucas
Arulkumaran Sabaratnam
*Harrow and London*

## CHAPTER 1

# Morbidity and mortality in the parturient

## Maternal mortality and CEMACH

The Confidential Enquiry into Maternal Deaths in England and Wales was launched in 1955. The report evolved into the Confidential Enquiry into Maternal and Child Health (CEMACH) which came into being on 1 April 2003. CEMACH, funded by the National Patient Safety Agency (NPSA), was an independent body with board members being made up of representatives from the Royal College of Obstetricians and Gynaecologists (RCOG), Midwives (RCM), Anaesthetists (RCA), Pathologists, Paediatrics and Child Health and the Faculty of Public Health Medicine of the Royal College of Physicians. The report is the longest running and most complete record of the causes of maternal death in the developed world. The reduction on maternal death rates not only in the UK but also throughout the world owes a huge debt to these triennial reports. On 1 July 2009, CEMACH became an independent charity with the new name 'Centre for Maternal and Child Enquiries' (CMACE).

The leading causes of maternal mortality are shown in Box 1.1.

The leading cause of direct maternal death in the UK is thrombosis and/or thromboembolic disease, and this has been the case for more than 20 years. However, within this group the pattern of disease has changed over this period. There has been a decrease in the number of deaths due to pulmonary embolism after caesarean section, almost certainly as a result of increased awareness in the obstetric team and meticulous use of thromboprophylaxis guidelines. This pattern has not been reflected in the number of antepartum deaths where there has been a slight increase since 1985.

---

*Handbook of Obstetric High Dependency Care*, 1st edition. By © D. Vaughan, N. Robinson, N. Lucas and S. Arulkumaran. Published 2010 by Blackwell Publishing Ltd

Box 1.1  Causes of maternal mortality in the UK
(CEMACH 2003–2005)

**Direct**
- Thrombosis/thromboembolic disease (TED)
- Pre-eclampsia/eclampsia
- Amniotic fluid embolism
- Genital tract sepsis
- Haemorrhage

**Indirect**
- Cardiac disease
- Psychiatric disease

Genital tract sepsis has again become a leading cause of maternal death in the UK and this is of particular relevance to the maternity high dependency unit (MHDU) where it is likely that not only women with a diagnosis of sepsis may be cared for but also women who are at risk of maternal sepsis. It was commented upon in the last confidential enquiry that the advent of antibiotics and aseptic precautions had led to a dramatic reduction in the number of deaths from sepsis in the early years of the confidential enquiry and that this in turn had removed the anxiety of maternal sepsis from our 'collective memory'. The report recommended action to raise awareness of the recognition and management of maternal sepsis in all healthcare professionals who may care for the obstetric patient and also that maternal early warning scoring systems be implemented.

Cardiac disease is now the leading overall cause of maternal death in the UK. The principal causes of death in this group are aortic dissection and myocardial ischaemia. The changes over the last 50 years in the population of women of childbearing age in the UK (rising maternal age at childbirth, increasing levels of obesity) are likely to have had an impact in this area.

Despite the huge impact of the report, the UK maternal mortality rate has not fallen in recent years (Figure 1.1). A number of factors may have contributed to this lack of decline. One possible explanation for this is the increasing numbers of high risk patients becoming pregnant.

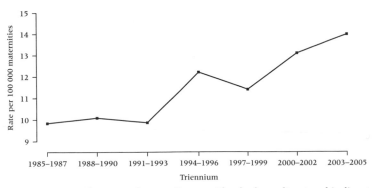

**Figure 1.1** Overall maternal mortality rate (deaths from direct and indirect causes combined) per 100 000 maternities, UK, CEMACH.

## Maternal morbidity

There is increasing recognition of the importance of the relationship between mortality and morbidity. Unlike maternal mortality, the full extent of maternal morbidity is not known. In a case control study published by Waterstone et al. (2001) estimated the incidence of severe obstetric morbidity at 12.0/100 deliveries. Another study from the USA estimated that 43% of women experienced some form of maternal morbidity.

Women who have experienced and survived a severe health condition in the antepartum period, at delivery or in the postpartum period are considered as cases of 'near miss' or 'severe acute maternal morbidity' (SAMM). The terms 'near miss' and 'SAMM' have been used interchangeably but the World Health Organization (WHO) working group on maternal morbidity and mortality recommends the use of the term 'maternal near miss'. There are various definitions of maternal near miss and these have been amalgamated by the WHO to provide one clear definition (Box 1.2).

**Box 1.2** WHO International Statistical Classification of Diseases and Related Health Problems, 10th Revision (ICD10) – Definition of maternal near miss

A woman who nearly died but survived a complication during pregnancy, childbirth or within 42 days of termination of the pregnancy

In the past, maternal mortality and morbidity have been studied in isolation from one another, but it is clear that if the two are treated as separate clinical entities and by only investigating mortality, the chance to detect other problems in maternity care is lost. The relationship between morbidity and mortality in pregnancy has been described as a 'continuum of adverse pregnancy events' (Box 1.3).

---

**Box 1.3** The continuum of adverse pregnancy events

Normal healthy pregnancy → Morbidity → Severe Morbidity → Near miss → Death

*Source*: Stacie E Geller. Am J Obstet Gynecol 2004;191:939–944.

---

Studies into maternal near miss cases have shown that the predominant underlying obstetric causes of obstetric morbidity differ somewhat from the major causes of maternal mortality. In the most recent CEMACH report, haemorrhage was the fourth commonest cause of direct maternal death, but in the Scottish audit of obstetric morbidity it was by far the most common cause of obstetric morbidity. Therefore it has been suggested that while enquiries into maternal near misses cannot completely act as a surrogate for maternal mortality, they can deliver information that complements the findings of studies into maternal deaths. What is perhaps even more interesting is the fact that it has been shown that a woman's progression along the continuum is affected by medical decision-making. This would suggest that identification of the high risk parturient as early as possible should have a major role in the primary and secondary prevention of morbidity and mortality.

## Maternal mortality, morbidity and the MHDU

The purpose of an MHDU is to provide care to women at risk of or experiencing morbidity at any stage during the antenatal or postnatal period. It is required to improve care and reduce maternal mortality and morbidity for the sick or high risk obstetric patient. There are two major components of MHDU care (Box 1.4).

---

**Box 1.4** Major components of maternity high dependency care

• Timely recognition of the sick or high risk obstetric patient
• Delivery of high quality, dedicated maternity high dependency care

## The high risk parturient

The term 'high risk' in association with pregnancy is often used interchangeably to refer to either the mother *or* the fetus being high risk. For the purposes of this discussion, the term 'high risk parturient' refers to a pregnant woman at risk of developing serious morbidity or mortality. Factors that may put a woman into the high risk parturient group may be divided into four categories (Box 1.5).

---

**Box 1.5**  Factors that may predispose a parturient to becoming high risk

**Pre-existing disease**
- Heart disease – congenital, ischaemic, valvular
- Respiratory disease – asthma, cystic fibrosis
- Renal – acute or chronic renal failure
- Neurological – e.g. multiple sclerosis, epilepsy, cerebrovascular disease
- Musculoskeletal – e.g. scoliosis ± surgery, connective tissue disorders
- Haematological – thrombocytopenia, thrombophilias

**Pregnancy-related disease**
- Pre-eclampsia
- Haemorrhage
- Acute fatty liver
- Peri-partum cardiomyopathy

**Social factors**
- Social disadvantage
- Poor communities
- Ethnic minorities
- Late bookers
- Obesity
- Domestic violence
- Substance abuse

**Miscellaneous factors**
- Jehovah's witness
- Needle phobia
- Anaesthetic-related issues – e.g. allergy, suxamethonium apnoea

---

# Identification of the high risk parturient

Identification of the 'high risk' parturient is key to the prevention of obstetric morbidity and mortality. Early identification allows time to plan effective multidisciplinary management strategies for the high risk woman. It is the responsibility of all healthcare professionals who may be (but not necessarily routinely) involved in the care of the pregnant woman. A woman may be identified as being high risk at any stage from pre-conception through to the booking visit, antenatal appointments, labour and the puerperium. The assessment of risk should take place at every opportunity.

## Points of referral

### Multidisciplinary antenatal clinics and the obstetric anaesthesia antenatal clinic

The schedule for antenatal care in the UK has been clearly laid out by National Institute for Clinical Excellence (NICE). The guideline refers to care of the healthy pregnant woman but within the algorithm it does highlight woman who may need additional care (Box 1.6).

> **Box 1.6** Women needing additional care as specified by NICE guideline
>
> * Cardiac disease, including hypertension
> * Renal disease
> * Endocrine disorders or diabetes requiring insulin
> * Psychiatric disorders (being treated with medication)
> * Haematological disorders
> * Autoimmune disorders
> * Epilepsy requiring anticonvulsant drugs
> * Malignant disease
> * Severe asthma
> * Use of recreational drugs
> * Human immunodeficiency virus (HIV) or Hepatitis B virus (HBV) infection
> * Obesity (body mass index, BMI, 30 kg/m² or above)
> * Underweight (BMI below 18 kg/m²)
> * Higher risk of developing complications, e.g. women aged 40 and older
> * Women who smoke
> * Women who are particularly vulnerable (such as teenagers) or who lack social support

Women who need additional care should be seen in multi-disciplinary antenatal clinics. Multidisciplinary clinics ideally use a list of named physicians representing all specialities so that the obstetrician in charge of the case can contact the physician to review the case together and develop a management plan. The value of multi-disciplinary antenatal clinics to allow forward planning for patients who may be high risk has long been recognised. For example, National guidelines (Obstetric Anaesthetists Association/Association of Anaesthetists Guidelines for Obstetric Anaesthetic Services, Revised Edition, 2005) have stressed the importance of timely anaesthetic involvement in the management of high risk pregnancies. Increasingly, referral to these clinics has become an essential step in the care pathway of the high risk parturient. Early attendance of a high risk parturient at the multidisciplinary antenatal clinic confers a number of advantages (Box 1.7).

---

**Box 1.7** Rationale for high risk parturient attendance at multidisciplinary antenatal clinic

- Assessment of patient and potential to deteriorate; optimisation if required
- Consideration of possible peri-partum complications
- Allows for adequate time to obtain necessary investigations
- Improved patient/healthcare professional partnership; communication, informed decision-making
- Allows time for referral and advice from other disciplines, e.g. cardiologists
- Starting point for *written* management strategy for elective and emergency situations
- Good environment for teaching and training.

---

Development of these clinics requires significant input from trusts. Financial constraints are clearly one of the major factors that may limit the extension of this service in hospitals. It has been estimated that only 30% of units in the UK have a dedicated anaesthetic antenatal clinic. Many units still rely on *ad hoc* referrals between obstetricians and anaesthetists. When this is the case, it is essential that there are clear lines of communication between all specialist teams and the maternity unit.

### Labour ward
It has been suggested that up to 90% of non-elective caesarean sections could be predicted. Furthermore from critical care outreach

work in the general population, we know that cardiorespiratory arrest is almost always preceded by a period of physiological instability. Therefore in a labour ward setting, multidisciplinary ward rounds (obstetric, anaesthetic and midwifery) play an essential role in identifying the at-risk parturient.

## Ward referrals and maternal early warning scores (MEWS)

High risk clinics will not detect healthy pregnant women who develop unexpected complications of pregnancy. Early warning scores have been used in the general hospital population for several years. In the 2003–2005 CEMACH report, a key recommendation was that a national obstetric early warning chart, similar to those in use in other areas of clinical practice be developed for use in all obstetric women. More recently the Clinical Negligence Scheme for Trusts (CNSTs) revised standards for Maternity Clinical Risk Management (2009) has, as a level 1 requirement that a 'maternity service has an approved guideline/documentation which describes the process for ensuring the early recognition of severely ill pregnant women and prompt access to either a high dependency unit (HDU) or intensive care unit (ICU)'.

The confidential enquiry report suggested that in the absence of a national chart, hospitals should adopt one of the existing early warning scoring systems currently available. Currently there is no universally validated scoring system available for obstetrics.

An early warning system is essentially a track and trigger system. It uses data derived from different physiological readings (e.g. systolic blood pressure (BP), heart rate (HR), respiratory rate, body temperature, conscious level, urine output) to generate a score which above a certain level triggers a 'response'. Alternately, data is recorded on a chart that is 'colour coded to red, yellow or green'. The trigger would occur if one parameter fell into the red zone or two parameters fell into the yellow zone.

There are various potential difficulties associated with the development of a MEWS system. The first and most obvious is that the physiological changes of pregnancy mean that the charts in use for the general population would not be directly applicable to the pregnant woman. There are also concerns that by using a MEWS system for all pregnant women, there may be further overmedicalisation of the birthing process. Furthermore implementing a MEWS system for all women on the maternity unit would undoubtedly significantly increase workload in an area which is often already stretched to capacity. For example, the majority of suggested MEWS systems have respiratory rate as one of the measured variables. Respiratory rate cannot be measured with an automated system and therefore would undoubtedly impact on the nursing/midwifery workload on a ward. How then should one target an early warning system in the obstetric population? It does not seem logical to limit it to women who have already been identified as being high risk or who have suffered a complication of pregnancy (e.g. post-partum haemorrhage) alone as these individuals have already been 'flagged-up'. Therefore it would seem sensible to extend its use to a subgroup of women who may be at risk of becoming 'high risk.' In addition the CEMACH report has suggested that these systems be used for pregnant women being cared for outside the obstetric setting, e.g. in gynaecology wards and accident and emergency departments. A list of suggested at-risk groups to include for MEWS monitoring are shown in Box 1.8.

---

**Box 1.8** Suggested at-risk groups suitable for MEWS monitoring

Post-operatively, e.g. lower segment caesarean section (LSCS)
Any woman who has had a spinal/epidural/patient-controlled analgesia (PCA)
Post-partum haemorrhage
Antepartum haemorrhage
Women with raised BP
Severe pre-eclampsia/eclampsia
Women with diabetes
Women with pre-labour rupture of membranes >24h
Any suspected or diagnosed infection
Women receiving oxygen or with an oxygen saturation ($SaO_2$) of <94%
Women undergoing blood transfusion
Post-intensive treatment unit (ITU)/HDU patients
Any woman who is readmitted after discharge from post-natal wards
Any pregnant woman admitted via the accident and emergency department
Any midwifery or medical concern

---

Of equal importance to the early recognition of patients with potential or established critical illness is the timely attendance to all such patients by those who possess appropriate skills, knowledge and experience. The CEMACH report has stated that 'detection of life-threatening illness alone is of little value; it is the subsequent management that will alter the outcome'. If these systems are to be adopted it is essential that enough resources are available, particularly with regard to staff training, in the places where they are to be used (including non-obstetric settings such as accident and emergency departments).

Other questions that remain to be answered and should be considered in the development of a MEWS system include how frequently should a patient undergo MEWS scoring and also for what time period MEWS scoring should be continued in any one patient?

The use of MEWS is not a substitute for sound clinical judgement nor do they mandate immediate HDU/ICU admission for the patient whose score has 'triggered' the second part of the system. Evidence from work in the non-obstetric population has not demonstrated that they act as either predictors of the development of critical illness or overall outcome from critical illness. What MEWS almost certainly do offer is an aid to effective communication between all members of the clinical team by acting as a common language.

The basic requirements for development of a MEWS system are shown in Box 1.9.

---

**Box 1.9** MEWS systems – basic requirements for development

Parameters – systolic blood pressure (SBP), HR, respiratory rate, body temperature, conscious level, urine output
Trigger – numerical or colour coded
Response to trigger – develop local algorithm encompassing
• immediate treatment measures
• investigations required
• escalation procedure – who to call
Further monitoring and review

---

### Post-natal care on the wards and in the community
Identification of the high risk parturient does not end when the woman has delivered and been discharged from hospital. This is particularly important for those women who have normal deliveries

and are rapidly discharged (6 h) from hospital. This also applies to women who deliver at home. In the 2000–2002 Confidential Enquiry, two women who had delivered at home died from puerperal sepsis.

The importance of good communication between the hospital, GP and community midwives has been highlighted, particularly if there have been any problems preceding/during the delivery. Although the use of MEWS may not be applicable in this setting, the importance of recording and acting upon any abnormality of basic observations (HR, BP and respiratory rate) cannot be under-estimated. Care of the post-natal patient must also include an assessment of the lochia. Lastly it cannot be emphasised enough that any patient with a temperature or who is unwell must be rapidly referred to hospital.

## CHAPTER 2

# The maternity high dependency unit

In the 1991–1993 Confidential Enquiry, the role of intensive care in the management of obstetric patients featured for the first time as a separate chapter and successive reports have made recommendations about the provision of adequate facilities to care for the 'high risk' parturient. The purpose of an MHDU is to provide care to women at risk of or experiencing morbidity at any stage during the ante-natal or post-natal period.

It may be difficult to distinguish between care provided between ICUs, HDUs and general wards as different hospitals will have different services available. However, a useful starting point comes from the review of adult critical care services by the department of health. This has recommended a classification of critically ill patients according to clinical need (Box 2.1).

---

**Box 2.1** Classification of critically ill patients

**Level 0**
Patients whose needs can be met through normal ward care in an acute hospital.

**Level 1**
Patients at risk of their condition deteriorating, or those recently relocated from higher levels of care whose needs can be met on an acute ward with additional advice and support from the critical care team.

*(Continued)*

---

*Handbook of Obstetric High Dependency Care*, 1st edition. By © D. Vaughan, N. Robinson, N. Lucas and S. Arulkumaran. Published 2010 by Blackwell Publishing Ltd

**Box 2.1** (Continued)

**Level 2**
Patients requiring more detailed observation or intervention including support for a single failing organ system or post-operative care, and those stepping down from higher levels of care.

**Level 3**
Patients requiring advanced respiratory support alone or basic respiratory support together with support of at least two organ systems. This level includes all complex patients requiring support for multi-organ failure.

Patients who require admission to an MHDU are likely to require Level 1 or 2 care, although some patients who require Level 2 care may need transfer to an ICU. The intensive care society (ICS) has further expanded this guidance to clarify exactly what may be expected of Levels 1 and 2 care (Box 2.2).

**Box 2.2** Intensive care society expanded guidance on levels of care

| *Level 1 criteria* | *Examples* |
| --- | --- |
| Patient recently discharged from a higher level of care | |
| Patients in need of additional monitoring, clinical input or advice | Observations required at least 4 hourly |
| Patients requiring critical care outreach service support | Abnormal vital signs but not requiring a higher level of care |
| Patients requiring staff with special expertise and/or additional facilities for at least one aspect of critical care delivered in a general ward environment | Epidural analgesia |

| Level 2 criteria | Examples |
|---|---|
| Patients needing single organ system monitoring and support | Respiratory – Needing more than 50% inspired oxygen |
| | Cardiovascular – Unstable requiring continuous electrocardiogram (ECG) and invasive pressure monitoring |
| Patients needing extended post-operative care | |

## Operational policy

A helpful and important component in the development of the MHDU is the operational policy that directs how the unit is actually going to run. As well as covering features such as admission/discharge criteria the operational policy should look at practical aspects of the MHDU (Box 2.3).

---

**Box 2.3** Components of operational policy for the MHDU

Philosophy and objectives of unit

Facilities
• Beds
• Bathrooms
• Clean and dirty utilities
• Desks/computers

Admission criteria

Discharge criteria

Staffing
• Medical/midwifery/nursing
• Roles of team members

Support services
• Other medical specialities, e.g. cardiology
• Physiotherapy
• Pharmacy
• Portering facilities

Guidelines/protocols and policies

Equipment

---

## Admission to the MHDU

The decision to admit a woman to the MHDU must involve the obstetric, midwifery and anaesthetic teams. If an admission occurs when a consultant obstetrician or anaesthetist is not immediately available, that consultant should be informed. The MHDU may also be used as an 'ICU step down' for an obstetric patient who has required admission to the ICU. A list of suggested admission criteria appear in Box 2.4. Ultimately, the decision to admit a patient should be based on clinical judgement. The suggested list is provided to assist but not be didactic or exclusive.

---

**Box 2.4** Suggested admission criteria for MHDU

- Transfer back from ICU, i.e. step down
- Moderate/severe pre-eclampsia
- Haemolysis, elevated liver enzymes and low platelets (HELLP) syndrome
- Obstetric haemorrhage
- Sickle crisis
- Diabetic stabilisation
- Women with suspected or diagnosed pulmonary embolus (PE)
- Asthma or compromised respiratory function
- Sepsis/suspected sepsis
- Any woman requiring intensive nursing or medical care

---

## Discharge from the MHDU

Women who have been cared for on the MHDU should be considered suitable for discharge when the disease process or physiological disturbance that led to the admission has been reversed. Suggested discharge criteria are shown in Box 2.5.

---

**Box 2.5** Suggested discharge criteria for the MHDU

- Patient is conscious and alert
- Stable and normal respiratory status
- Stable and normal haemodynamic parameters with no evidence of haemorrhage
- Intensive/invasive monitoring is no longer required and 4-hourly recording of vital signs is considered appropriate

In our unit we use a discharge sheet based on these criteria (Box 2.6).

---

**Box 2.6** Discharge sheet for all patients being transferred from MHDU*

|  | Tick |
|---|:---:|
| A – Airway: the patient can maintain their airway | ☐ |
| B – Breathing: respiratory rate and oxygen saturations are within normal limits and have been documented | ☐ |
| C – HR & BP normal, stable for four hours preceding discharge | ☐ |
| The patient is alert and orientated | ☐ |
| The uterus is well contracted and the lochia is normal Loss from surgical drains is acceptable | ☐ |
| The wound is clean and dry | ☐ |
| The patient is comfortable (*pain score is less than 3/10***) | ☐ |
| Patient has received treatment for post-operative nausea & vomiting | ☐ |
| The patient is apyrexial | ☐ |
| Intensive/invasive monitoring is no longer required and 4 hourly recording of vital signs is considered appropriate | ☐ |
| Anti-embolic stockings worn as per guidelines for thromboprophylaxis | ☐ |
| Drug chart has been reviewed by doctor and is accurate (with particular reference to DVT prophylaxis, if required, and antibiotics) | ☐ |
| Bed has been booked on the appropriate ward | ☐ |
| An on-going plan of care has been clearly written by the obstetrician | ☐ |
| There has been a verbal hand over to the receiving ward – midwife to midwife | ☐ |
| Midwife signature | Date |

ALL BOXES MUST BE TICKED BEFORE A PATIENT IS DISCHARGED

*This chart may also be useful for patients being discharged from obstetric recovery
**Aim for post caesarean section analgesia: >90% women to have a worst pain score of <3 on a VAS of 0–10.

*Source*: Raising the Standard: A Compendium of Audit Recipes, 2nd Edition, 2006.

## Transfer to ICU

Some patients on the MHDU may progress to requiring ICU care (Level 3 care). An underlying principle of admitting a patient to the ICU is that the patient should benefit from ICU care. There is good evidence in studies from the general population that delays in the transfer of critically ill patients to the ICU can significantly increase the mortality rate. Therefore it is essential that every unit has clear pathways in place to facilitate transfer to the ICU. There should be close cooperation between the MHDU and ICU teams at an early stage with consultant-to-consultant referral and early involvement of the ICU consultant and other specialities in specific situations (e.g. cardiology). Intensive care is a treatment and not a place and once it has been decided that a woman would benefit from ICU care, this care should be instigated immediately, e.g. a woman may require intubation and ventilation on the MHDU prior to transfer. Suggested criteria for women who may require escalation to ICU care are shown in Box 2.7.

---

**Box 2.7** Situations where a woman may require escalation of care from the MHDU to ICU

Women who require ventilatory support, invasive/non-invasive*
Women who require cardiovascular organ support with inotropes
Women with multi-organ failure

*Some MHDUs may be able to offer non-invasive ventilatory support.

---

For some stand-alone units transferring a patient to ICU may require an inter-hospital transfer. The ICS has published guidelines for the transport of the critically ill patient covering all aspects of inter- and intra-hospital transfer. The key points of these guidelines are summarised in Box 2.8.

Within the ICS guidelines there are helpful appendices with checklists covering aspects of the patient's preparation for transfer, equipment checks and documentation.

## Personnel

MHDUs are increasingly becoming an integral part of any large hospital-based labour ward. The Association of Anaesthetists/Obstetric

---

**Box 2.8** Key components of safe patient transfer to an ICU

**Preparation**
- Close liaison between HDU and ICU teams
- Patient is meticulously resuscitated and stabilised prior to transfer

**Equipment**
- Monitoring – the standard of monitoring should be at least as good as that on the MHDU. Minimum standards include ECG, non-invasive blood pressure, arterial saturation, end tidal carbon dioxide in ventilated patients, temperature. Monitoring should be continuous throughout the transfer and easily visible
- Ventilator – adequate oxygen supply, disconnection/high pressure alarms, ability to control inspired oxygen concentration

**Personnel**
- A minimum of two trained accompanying attendants, e.g. anaesthetist/intensivist and midwife

**Practical aspects**
- Safety of the patient – suitable trolley with patient safely secured
- Warming – warm air devices, blankets, patient dignity ensured at all times
- Mode of transport

**Communication**
- Note keeping – written records maintained throughout transfer
- Handover – verbal and written account of patients' history, vital signs and ongoing treatment between transfer and receiving staff

---

Anaesthetists Association guidelines for obstetric anaesthesia services state that 'high dependency care should be available on or near the delivery suite with appropriately-trained staff'. One of the biggest challenges facing any unit developing a MHDU is the issue of staffing.

## Medical

There are no clear guidelines available about the most appropriate way to provide medical cover to the MHDU. The obvious candidates are either members of the obstetric or anaesthetic teams although there are inherent difficulties with both groups in this context. Obstetricians will have expert knowledge of the particular problems of the parturient; however, with the advent of run-through training they may have had little or no training in areas of acute medicine outside obstetrics. Anaesthetists may have greater knowledge of the management of an acutely ill patient but altering their role to become that of obstetric HDU physicians would have a major impact on the delivery of analgesia in labour and anaesthesia for caesarean section. What is clear is that each unit must agree a strategy that provides adequate medical supervision to the MHDU at all times (including weekends). A practical solution would be for obstetricians to continue to care for their patients including those on the maternity HDU with significant input from the anaesthesia team (multidisciplinary wards rounds).

## Midwifery/Nursing

Labour wards are predominantly staffed by midwives with support from midwifery assistants and in some units nursing staff. It would seem logical to draw upon midwives to staff an HDU, and to a large extent midwives are ideally placed to take on the role of caring for MHDU patients. This extension of the midwives' role has been recognised by the Royal College of Midwives, who in the guidance published in January 2006 stated that midwives are increasingly being asked to 'extend and enhance the scope of their professional practice to address the challenges of modern obstetric care'. MHDU care is clearly an area that falls into this category. However, midwifery staff who have largely been concerned with the care of the parturient may be unfamiliar with the needs of and particular skills required to care for the MHDU patient. Midwives who have trained through the direct entry programme may be further disadvantaged in this context. Another option that could be considered to staff the MHDU is to draw staff from a general nursing background. However, this is not ideal either as using staff from a purely nursing background ignores the particular needs of pregnant women who suffer a complication of pregnancy and become 'patients'. The RCM guidance states that 'the RCM strongly recommends that the developments of new practices or reallocated responsibilities are set in the context of improved quality and continuity of care' and that further training and education are necessary to equip midwifery staff for this new activity. In our unit, the MHDU is staffed with a combination of midwifery staff and nursing staff from a general medical background. Midwifery and nursing staff are required to attend a mandatory training week on all aspects of working on the labour ward. In addition we run a training day about care of the MHDU patient.

A further consideration with regard to midwifery/nursing staff on the MHDU is the unpredictability of admissions to the MHDU. The Obstetric Anaesthetists Association (OAA)/Association of Anaesthetists of Great Britain and Ireland (AAGBI) guidelines states that when high dependency care is required, the midwife/nurse-to-patient ratio must be at least one midwife/nurse to two patients and that appropriately trained staff should be available 24 hours per day. Some units may choose to work with a team of HDU-trained midwives while others may try to ensure that the majority of staff are able to work in the MHDU with appropriate support when required. We have found the latter option helpful in our unit.

## Documentation and record keeping

It is essential to good medical practice and as an intrinsic part of risk management that documentation relating to a patient's care is of the highest standard. This includes the medical notes, nursing/midwifery charts, anaesthetic charts and drug charts. In the MHDU it is likely that more than one specialty may be involved in the care of the woman. It is essential that these teams not only communicate closely with one another but that records of each visit and changes or additions to the management are recorded meticulously. We have found it helpful to have a minimum dataset of daily standards for the MHDU (Box 2.9).

---

**Box 2.9** Minimum standards for MHDU patients' daily review

**Examination**
Pyrexia?

*Respiratory system (RS)*
Respiratory rate
Oxygen saturation and inspired oxygen concentration (e.g. air, 2L)
Auscultation of the chest must be undertaken

*(Continued)*

**Box 2.9** (Continued)

*Cardiovascular system (CVS)*
Heart rate and blood pressure
Assessment of peripheral circulation in relevant patients, e.g.
massive obstetric haemorrhage

*Abdomen*
Soft?
No areas of tenderness/guarding
Bowel sounds present?

*Genitourinary (GU) system*
Urine output

*Central nervous system (CNS)*
Conscious?
Orientated?
Motor and sensory function of legs

*Obstetric specific observations*
• Wound
• Uterus
• Lochia

The results of all investigations should be checked at least once daily
and recorded in a flow chart.

An MHDU chart that clearly displays all the required observations,
blood results, ongoing therapy (including intravenous (IV) fluids and
drugs) is extremely useful for all clinicians caring for the patient.
A chart that is compatible with other high dependency areas in the
hospital (e.g. ICU) is ideal.

## Protocols and guidelines

A guideline is a document written to provide guidance on the
management of medical conditions or practice in a particular
medical setting (e.g. the MHDU). Protocols have the same function
as guidelines but may be more specific to individual conditions.
The aim of guidelines and protocols is to standardise and improve
care for patients at a local, national and international level. They

are an essential part of modern obstetric care with the impetus for their development coming from many organisations including the Confidential Enquiry, the RCOG, the RCA, the RCM and the OAA. Significantly for trusts they are a requirement at all CNST levels. Many of the labour ward protocols that are in existence will be directly applicable to the MHDU (e.g. pre-eclampsia, management of obstetric haemorrhage). A list of MHDU-specific guidelines is shown in Box 2.10.

---

**Box 2.10** MHDU-specific guidelines

Admission criteria
Discharge criteria
Criteria for the transfer of patients who require ICU care
Guideline for the use of invasive monitoring

---

## Environment and equipment

The MHDU should be a designated area for the care of the obstetric HDU patient on or very near the delivery suite. It should only be used for the care of the MHDU patient and should be equipped, maintained and have an appropriate skill mix of staff available at all times. Extending its use to that of a triage area, post-natal overflow or an area for woman having induction of labour devalues the concept of high dependency care and should not occur.

A suggested list of equipment for the MHDU is shown in Box 2.11.

---

**Box 2.11** Suggested equipment list for MHDU

Monitor for P, BP, ECG, $SaO_2$ and with transducer facility for invasive monitoring
Equipment for insertion and management of invasive monitoring (arterial and central venous pressure (CVP))
Piped oxygen and suction
IV fluid warmer
Forced air warming device
Blood gas analyser*

*(Continued)*

**Box 2.11** (Continued)

Infusion pumps
Emergency massive haemorrhage trolley*
Emergency eclampsia box*
Transfer equipment – monitor and ventilator
Computer terminal to facilitate access to blood results, picture archiving and communication system (PACS)
Copy of hospital obstetric guidelines (if not available on hospital intranet)
Resuscitation trolley with defibrillator and airway management equipment

*These items may already be available in theatres on delivery suite.

## Clinical governance, audit and risk management

Clinical governance is the generic term for the multiple processes involved in the maintenance and development of high standards in patient care. Effective clinical governance encompassing clinical audit, education and training, risk management and research and development are fundamental aspects of modern obstetric care. Their relevance is emphasised in the CNST standards.

In January 2008 the RCOG published guidance on the 'maternity dashboard – a clinical performance and governance score card'. The maternity dashboard is a tool that can be used to monitor the implementation of principles of clinical governance. It can be used to monitor performance against locally agreed standards and also to allow comparison between units. In the same way a car dashboard provides information about its function (fuel, speed, etc.), the maternity 'dashboard' aims to provide information about the functioning of the maternity unit. The four categories of parameters that should be included on the maternity dashboard are:
• Clinical activity
• Workforce
• Clinical outcomes
• Risk incidents/complaints
As well as the data that is collected a traffic light system is used to highlight areas of concern with upper and lower thresholds.

- Green – when goals are met
- Amber – when the goals are not met but activity is still above the lower threshold
- Red – when the goals are not met and activity is below the lower threshold (immediate action required)

Activity within the MHDU must be included in a hospitals' maternity dashboard. It is likely that in most hospitals using the maternity dashboard markers of maternal morbidity necessitating HDU admission already appear. With the development of MHDUs it would be useful to also include MHDU-specific midwife/patient ratios, outcomes as demonstrated by discharge environment (e.g. ward versus ICU) and critical incidents on the MHDU.

## The MHDU patient and ethical challenges

The fundamental tenet of modern obstetric care is the care should be woman centred and those women, their partners and families should be treated with kindness, respect and dignity at all times. It is intrinsic to this a woman's views and beliefs should be respected. In obstetric situations the ethical issues largely focus on the maternal fetal relationship but in the MHDU setting this may not always be the predominant issue. Furthermore when a pregnant/recently delivered woman becomes ill the first priority is her physical well being. However, recognising and caring for the impact of the physical disease on her emotional well being is also extremely important. Failure to care for a woman in this regard may put her at risk of post-traumatic stress disorder after the event which may have serious effects on maternal bonding.

**PART I**
# Emergency care

## CHAPTER 3

# Emergency management of the obstetric patient – general principles

Advances in obstetric, neonatal and general medical care over the last two decades along with major and ongoing changes in population demographics and social behaviour have resulted in a significant change in activity on and around the delivery suite. Women who in the past would never have had children are now able to do so, and present with significant congenital or acquired co-morbidities. Similarly the understanding and management of both obstetric and general medical conditions has improved to a point where maternal morbidity is regarded now as a disastrous aberration rather than inevitable. All of these factors (see Box 3.1) increase demand on maternity services in general and high dependency facilities in particular.

**Box 3.1** Factors contributing to increasing complexity of patient care

- Aging maternity population
- Increasing complexity of coexistent disease
- Higher standards of monitoring
- Increasing numbers of therapies and intervention
- Increasing healthcare expectations from patients, relatives, professional bodies, the state and the courts
- Reduced medical and nursing/midwifery staffing and experience, increased handover and cross-cover

*Handbook of Obstetric High Dependency Care*, 1st edition. By © D. Vaughan, N. Robinson, N. Lucas and S. Arulkumaran. Published 2010 by Blackwell Publishing Ltd

The capacity of a mother to withstand the rigours and physiological demands of pregnancy and delivery depends on her physiological reserve and the stress placed upon it during this process. The challenge of dealing with patients with impaired reserve is the *raison d'être* of obstetric high dependency care, and depends on three mechanisms working together (Box 3.2) to allow the early identification and correction of complications.

---

**Box 3.2** Complimentary approaches to high dependency care

1 **P**rediction – identification of an at-risk population
2 **P**revention
3 **P**rompt identification of and intervention in complications

---

This chapter seeks to outline the general principles of assessment and management when confronted with an unstable patient, although it is a good system to apply to review on any complicated case. The emphasis is on logical and systematic review, planning and treatment. There are several excellent courses run by the Royal Colleges of Obstetrics and Gynaecology and of Surgery, which provide practical experience of system application. We would particularly recommend the CCrISP course (Care of the Critically Ill Surgical Patient, Royal College of Surgeons, RCS) as a good generic guide to the management of all unstable or complex patients.

The approach to management is outlined below. An initial swift assessment is designed to eliminate or detect life-threatening emergencies and gather information. This is followed by a more detailed review of the patient, their charts, notes, etc., and then planning and action (Box 3.3). More detailed descriptions of

---

**Box 3.3** Generic management plan

*Immediate assessment*
ABCDE
↓
*Full patient assessment*
Chart and note review, systems exam, investigations
↓
*Decisions and planning*
*Stable* → management plan
*Unstable/unsure* → diagnosis required; investigations/referral

---

the management of specific conditions are found in later chapters of this book.

## Immediate assessment

This process prioritises the order in which assessments and treatment are carried out, although in reality much of this is done simultaneously. A satisfactory reply to 'Hello, how are you feeling' tells us that the patient has a clear airway, good enough respiratory function to speak normally and oxygenate her blood such that her adequately functioning CVS can perfuse her brain, and that her central nervous system is functioning well enough to generate a socially appropriate reply. This doesn't abrogate responsibility for a full assessment, but it is a classic example of how much information can be simply and quickly gained.

Immediate assessment is based on a swift but careful ABCDE, using a 'look, listen, feel, treat' approach. ANY evidence of a significant problem will require more than one trained staff member to correct – so call for help earlier rather than later. In the routine review of a mother on the obstetric HDU, the immediate assessment in the presence of normal observations or as part of a planned ward round is still important but may well be more cursory in nature, and included in the general introductions to establish identity and rapport with the patient. In the unstable patient it is important to use appropriate monitoring (electrocardiograph, blood pressure and pulse oximetry as a minimum) as soon as is practical if not already present and attached.

### A – Airway

Without a clear airway, breathing is not possible, hence this comes first. Assessment is swift and simple (Box 3.4). Although unlikely in the MHDU setting, it is important to note that in cases where

---

**Box 3.4** Airway

**Look** – cyanosis, obstructed/see-saw respiratory pattern, increased respiratory work, tracheal tug, obvious airway obstruction (vomit, foreign body)

**Listen** – abnormal sounds (stridor, hoarseness, gurgling, snoring, grunting)

**Feel** – inspiratory and expiratory air flow

*(Continued)*

---

**Box 3.4** (Continued)

**Treat** – immediate goal is to clear and secure the airway to prevent hypoxic damage to mother and child. Administer high flow oxygen (15 l/min oxygen, ideally via a rebreathing mask) and carry out simple manoeuvres to clear airway if obstructed – suction, jaw thrust, chin lift, insertion of Guedel airway. Failure of these manoeuvres is rare but will require anaesthetic intervention – try to maintain oxygenation whilst you wait for help with the above or bag/mask ventilation

---

trauma is suspected or cannot be excluded, airway management also includes in-line cervical spine immobilisation by hand until appropriate collars/sandbags can be applied or the cervical spine clinically and radiologically cleared.

## B – Breathing

Again, what is needed is not a gold medal winning assessment for whispering pectoriloquy but a swift and thorough check (Box 3.5).

---

**Box 3.5** Breathing

**Look** – cyanosis; rate, depth, pattern and equality of breathing; check oxygen saturation (remember, whilst this will tell you if the patient is hypoxic, it does NOT reflect the adequacy of ventilation in terms of carbon dioxide clearance). If chest drain(s) have been sited, check if bubbling, swinging or non-functional, and check drainage quantity and type (blood, serous, etc.).

**Listen** – ability to talk clearly and in sentences, cough, breathing noises. Percussion – note change; auscultation – abnormal breath sounds, also heart sounds and rhythm

**Treat** – clearly, this will depend on the cause found. During immediate assessment you should look for and treat life-threatening conditions (tension pneumothorax, cardiac tamponade, haemothorax) as well as considering severe asthma, bronchial obstruction, pulmonary blood or amniotic fluid embolism and cardiac failure

---

## C – Circulation

Hypovolaemia should always be considered as the primary cause of circulatory failure in the pregnant or recently delivered woman until proven otherwise, and haemorrhage (overt or covert) should be excluded or aggressively treated (see Box 3.6). Unless there are obvious signs of cardiogenic shock, any mother who is tachycardic and cool peripherally or hypotensive should be assumed to have hypovolaemic shock, should have at least 1 × 16G or larger cannula sited, have blood for urgent cross-match sent and be given a 10 ml/kg IV fluid bolus if normotensive and 20 ml/kg if hypotensive.

---

**Box 3.6** Circulation

**Look** – reduced peripheral perfusion (cold hand/feet, pallor, poor pulse oximeter trace), blood in bed/on pad/in drains; swollen abdomen
**Feel** – pulses (rate, quality)
**Treat** – establish monitoring, send blood for cross-match. Remember to use a lumbar wedge if the woman is antenatal to prevent aortocaval compression. Treatment is aimed at maintaining tissue oxygenation and perfusion, but remember that ONGOING haemorrhage will only be cured by surgical or radiological intervention. If antenatal remember fetal monitoring as placental perfusion is dependent on maternal blood pressure – urgent delivery may be necessary

---

Hypovolaemic patients should always be regularly reassessed. Those who have a rapid, adequate and stable response to fluid resuscitation should be observed carefully. Those in whom resuscitation needs are ongoing will need rapid and definitive treatment, usually surgery. If any doubt exists as to the status of these patients, senior support should be sought early and rapidly. Major haemorrhage protocols are best activated early in obstetrics to ensure supply of blood and blood products.

## D – Disability/CNS dysfunction

In a primary survey this is a swift assessment to act as a future reference point if necessary (Box 3.7). Altered conscious level

> **Box 3.7** AVPU and pupil CNS function scoring
>
> **A** – alert
> **V** – responding to verbal stimulus
> **P** – responding to pain only
> **U** – unresponsive
> **Pupils** – size, equal left and right, response to bright light

can be due to many things in the obstetric population other than eclampsia! Hypoxia, hypercarbia, drug effects and primary cerebral events should also be considered. Bedside blood glucose (BM) estimation should be performed to exclude severe hypo- or hyperglycaemia.

### E – Exposure

Whilst the dignity and body temperature of a patient should be respected and protected wherever possible, adequate access for examination and intervention are vital. Change the patient into a gown to allow access and curtain off the treatment area if possible and practical. Consider a warming blanket if prolonged exposure is likely or the patient feels cold.

At the end of the initial assessment you should have a monitored patient, on oxygen and with IV access and fluid running. Baseline bloods (full blood count (FBC), U&Es, group and save as a minimum; ± cross-match, clotting, complement reactive protein (CRP), urate, blood cultures and anything else appropriate to the particulars of the case) should be on the way to the laboratory.

Your patient should be showing signs of improvement, and your help should be on the way or have arrived. Reassessment of any abnormalities found is vital and should be ongoing to check that your interventions are working. Now is the time to organise any pressing investigations you feel appropriate (blood gases, ECG, chest radiograph (CXR), catheterisation, fetal blood sampling, etc.). Whilst you wait for these interventions to work, this is a good time to continue to the next stage of assessment to establish the underlying cause of deterioration. If the patient continues to deteriorate despite your interventions as above, urgent transfer to ITU/theatre may well be necessary with ongoing resuscitation in the intervening period.

## Full patient assessment

### Note and chart review
A brief review of charts provides much information both from absolute values and trends. General factors are clearly important but attention should focus on those areas relevant to the individual cases (e.g. pre-eclamptic patient – blood pressure, urine output, drug infusions, urate and platelet values and *trends in these variables*). A systematic approach can make the interpretation of large amounts of data easier (Box 3.8).

---

**Box 3.8**  Chart assessment system

**Respiratory** – rate, oxygen requirement (inspired oxygen concentration, $FiO_2$), oxygen saturation ($SaO_2$)
**Circulatory** – Heart rate and rhythm, blood pressure, CVP
**Renal/Fluids** – Urine output, fluid balance
**Obstetric** – clearly patient specific, but also temperature, cardiotocogram (CTG), drains, reflexes, etc.
**Drugs** – prescribed drugs and doses. Given? Appropriate route?

---

Note review will highlight areas of concern and previous management plans or decisions. It will also provide information on co-morbidities, medications allergies and other factors often overlooked but of potentially vital importance.

### Systems examination
A full and thorough examination should now be performed, both to assess progress of any earlier interventions and to assess more fully the patient.

### Investigation/results review
Check through recent investigations, referring to current charts as necessary. Most HDUs use flow charts so that trends in haematological and biochemical variables can be tracked. Chase up outstanding radiological and microbiological investigations and reports.

## Decisions and planning

You should now be in a position, in consultation with the others involved in the patient's care, to decide if the patient is or remains stable. If this is the case formulate, agree and document a management plan. Remember to explain this to colleagues AND TO THE PATIENT. Document this clearly in the notes as well as the planned scope and time of the next review (Box 3.9).

---

**Box 3.9** Writing your summary

**Details** (patient name and number, date and time, your name and contact details)
**Assessment** – summary of events; clinical situation at present; treatment initiated and effect
**Management Plan** – investigations, interventions, drugs, nutrition, etc.
**Communication** – to patient/relatives/other staff
**Review** – planned; what parameter changes will necessitate earlier review

---

If you are unsure if the patient is stable, or if the patient is clearly not stable, determine what needs to be done to correct this. Further planning at this stage will usually necessitate the involvement of senior medical staff. At all times ensure the level of ongoing support and monitoring is appropriate for the patient (remember, a trip to the radiology department may yield more information but it is away from a critical care area and thus inherently more dangerous). Ensure your assessment and plans are recorded as well as a differential diagnosis and what you intend to do to move treatment on. Establish safe parameters for the patient and for future review.

## Invasive monitoring in the MHDU

Invasive monitoring can be used to more accurately monitor a patient's physiological parameters. The commonest two types of invasive monitoring that are used to monitor a patient's haemodynamic status in the HDU or ICU settings are arterial lines and central lines (sometimes referred to as central venous pressure or 'CVP' lines). These may both be used in the MHDU patient.

### Arterial lines
An arterial line is a cannula placed in a peripheral artery. The major indications for the insertion of an arterial line are shown in Box 3.10.

> **Box 3.10** Indications for insertion of arterial line
>
> • To enable measurement of blood pressure continuously
> • To enable the measurement of arterial blood gases and acid base status
> • To facilitate blood sampling in a patient requiring multiple blood tests negating the need for multiple venepuncture

Assessment of blood pressure is particularly important in the MHDU/critically ill patient. An arterial line with transducer enables the continuous assessment of blood pressure therefore allowing the immediate effects of medication to be seen, e.g. when using IV antihypertensives in pre-eclampsia.

The commonest site for insertion of a peripheral arterial line is the left or right radial artery, although the posterior tibial artery, dorsalis pedis and femoral arteries may all be used.

Arterial pressure may be measured from an arterial line using a transducer system. The transducer is fixed at the level of the right atrium of the patient and connected to the patient's arterial line via fluid-filled extension tubing connected to a bag of normal saline pressurised to 300 mmHg. It is essential to make sure there is no air in the system. The transducer is also connected to the monitor (Figure 3.1).

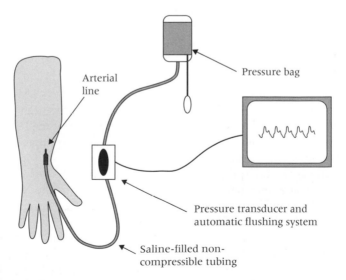

**Figure 3.1** Connections and set-up of invasive arterial monitor.

The transducer is 'zeroed' to atmospheric pressure by turning the three-way tap so that it is *open to the transducer and to room air, but closed to the patient*. A flat line should appear on the screen at this point. The three-way tap is then turned so that it is now closed to room air and open between the patient and the transducer. A continuous arterial trace reading should be visible on the screen.

## Central lines

A central line is a special type of venous cannula usually inserted into one of the great veins, most commonly the superior vena cava. The most common sites of insertion are the right or left internal jugular vein, the right or left subclavian vein or the femoral veins. Sometimes central lines are inserted via the antecubital fossa the elbow ('long lines').

The indications for central lines are shown in Box 3.11.

---

**Box 3.11**  Indications for insertion of central line

- To measure CVP and facilitate determination of volume status
- Administration of drugs, e.g. inotropic support with epinephrine
- To facilitate venous access in patients with poor peripheral access
- To facilitate blood sampling in patients requiring multiple blood tests

---

Central lines can be single lumen or multilumen. The most common sites for insertion are the internal jugular vein or the subclavian vein. They should only be inserted by trained individual, using a strict aseptic technique according to local guidelines. Contraindications to insertion of a central line include a patient with a known coagulopathy and this is of particular importance to the pre-eclamptic/eclamptic patient with deranged clotting in the MHDU. In this situation central venous access may be more safely obtained via a 'long line' inserted in the antecubital fossa.

In 2002 NICE issued guidance regarding the insertion of central lines which stated that ultrasound guidance should be the preferred method when inserting a central venous catheter into the internal jugular vein in adults and children in elective situations.

After insertion the correct position of the central line should be confirmed via X-ray.

CVP may be measured from a central line manually using a manometer system (intermittent readings, less accurate) or electronically using a transducer system (continuous readings, more accurate). The transducer system is the preferred method in the MHDU and the set-up is the same as for arterial lines. The transducer is fixed at the level of the right atrium of the patient and connected to the patient's central line via fluid-extension tubing connected to a bag of normal saline pressurised to 300 mmHg. The transducer is also connected to the monitor (see Figure 3.1). The transducer is 'zeroed' to atmospheric pressure by turning the three-way tap so that it is *open to the transducer and to room air, but closed to the patient*. A flat line should appear on the screen at this point. The three-way tap is then turned so that it is now closed to room air and open between the patient and the transducer. A continuous CVP reading should be visible on the screen.

As with all physiological parameters a single reading of CVP is less useful than a series of readings over time. Also the CVP should be used to assess the patient in conjunction with other haemodynamic variables (HR, BP, urine output).

## Care of arterial and central lines

It is essential that all types of invasive monitoring are managed according to local guidelines. Although potentially helpful in the management of the MHDU patient, their use does increase the risk of infection. It is essential that (1) they are inserted and cared for by trained practitioners and (2) any complications are detected and managed rapidly. The principles of care are summarised in Box 3.12.

---

**Box 3.12** Principles of care of invasive monitoring lines

- The date of insertion should be recorded
- Ensure all connections are secure
- Meticulous attention to correct position of three-way taps used in connections
- Arterial line/central line and connections should be *visible at all times*, not covered with blankets, etc.

*(Continued)*

**Box 3.12** (Continued)

• Arterial lines should be clearly labelled to reduce the risk of inadvertent drug administration through the arterial line
• Drug infusions through central lines should be clearly labelled
• All contact with invasive monitoring should be managed as aseptically as possible, e.g. sterile gloves, clean bungs

Invasive monitoring used in the MHDU setting is generally safe. However, there are potential risks which are summarised in Box 3.13.

**Box 3.13** Risks of invasive monitoring

**Central lines**
• Internal carotid artery puncture
• Pneumothorax/haemothorax
• Cardiac dysrhythmia
• Infection
• Air embolism

**Arterial lines**
• Thromboembolism/vasospasm/thrombosis
• Infection
• Damage to peripheral nerves
  – median, ulna, posterior tibial
• Local damage to artery itself
• Accidental intra-arterial injection of drugs
• Accidental disconnection and exsanguination

## CHAPTER 4
# Maternal and neonatal resuscitation

Staff in maternity units are unfamiliar with the management of maternal cardiac arrest. Despite regular training sessions, the anaesthetist tends to be regarded as the pivotal member of the maternal resuscitation team, and should take the lead when present. A dedicated registrar and senior house officer usually staff neonatal units in large centres. However, the paediatrician attending at deliveries is often the most junior, and thus it may fall to other staff members to assist in the early stages of neonatal resuscitation. All staff members should have a sound and up-to-date knowledge of basic and intermediate life support, as well as how to assist others when the appropriate crash team arrives.

## Maternal cardiac arrest

The cause of a cardiac arrest must be determined and all possible causes treated (see Box 4.1). There are two important features of maternal resuscitation which need to be carried out in addition to both basic and advanced life support (ALS). Firstly, cardiopulmonary resuscitation (CPR) will be unsuccessful if venous return is impaired and this occurs if the pregnant patient is resuscitated in the supine position. It is imperative that the cardiac arrest be managed with the patient in a partial left lateral position or using a 'human wedge' with the patient positioned in a left lateral tilt. This can be achieved by having an assistant kneel with their buttocks resting on their heels. The patient can than be propped over the thighs of the assistant and thus maintained in a stable, tilted position for CPR. Secondly, the baby needs to be delivered by caesarean

*Handbook of Obstetric High Dependency Care*, 1st edition. By © D. Vaughan, N. Robinson, N. Lucas and S. Arulkumaran. Published 2010 by Blackwell Publishing Ltd

> **Box 4.1** Causes of maternal cardiac arrest
>
> **Airway** – oedema, obstruction, misplaced or dislodged tube at general anaesthetic caesarean section
> **Breathing** – bronchospasm, pneumothorax
> **Circulatory** – cardiovascular collapse: *cardiogenic* (dysrhythmia, exacerbation of pre-existing condition, infarction, valvular disease); *septic* (chorioamnionitis, sepsis not related to pregnancy); *hypovolaemic* (haemorrhage, concealed/revealed, antepartum/post-partum)
> **Embolism** – clot (from deep vein thrombosis, DVT), amniotic fluid
> **Anaesthesia** – *epidural*, total spinal, intravenous injection; *general anaesthesia*, intubation problems, anaphylaxis, equipment/monitoring failure, malignant hyperpyrexia
> **Drugs** – Anaphylaxis
> **Cerebral** – bleeding, infection, infarction, seizure

section immediately. A well-managed maternal cardiac arrest should lead to the delivery of a live infant and improves the prospect of successful maternal outcome.

## Neonatal resuscitation

Most newborn babies establish respiration spontaneously after delivery, and the only care required initially is to dry and wrap the infant. Although deliveries in which a greater degree of support than this is required can be anticipated (see Box 4.2), fetal problems are often sudden and unexpected, so all should be familiar with the resuscitation equipment and protocol. It is vital

> **Box 4.2** Prenatal predictors of a need for fetal resuscitation
>
> Fetal distress
> Meconium-stained amniotic fluid (particularly if thick and fresh)
> Abnormal antenatal scans
> Abnormal presentation
> Multiple delivery
> Preterm delivery

to remember that the theatre team have a primary ethical and legal concern for the mother. If assisting in the neonatal resuscitation potentially jeopardises the mother (e.g. active bleeding), the scrub and anaesthetic team must *not* get involved with the care of a second patient.

Apgar scoring (see Box 4.3) is the most commonly used system for neonatal assessment. It is quick and provides a clear guide to the status of the fetus. It is routinely recorded at 1 and 5 min post-delivery. Any child who has a reduced Apgar score at delivery (i.e. less than 10/10) should be urgently assessed and treated appropriately.

---

**Box 4.3** Neonatal Apgar scores

| Clinical sign | Score | | |
|---|---|---|---|
| | 0 | 1 | 2 |
| Heart rate (beats per minute) | No pulse | <100 | >100 |
| Respiratory effort | Apnoea | Poor | Good |
| Colour (mucous membranes) | White | Blue | Pink |
| Muscle tone | Flaccid | Poor | Normal |
| Response to stimulation | None | Grimace | Cry |

---

## Airway

The optimum position of the neonatal airway differs from the 'sniffing the morning air' position in the adult because of the large size of the head in general and occiput in particular compared to the body. The infant should be flat on its back with the neck extended. Modern paediatric resuscitaires have a sloped leading edge to facilitate this position. If breathing does not commence immediately, gently reposition the child and suck out any mucus, fluid or meconium present from the mouth, nose or pharynx.

## Breathing

The first breath a baby takes is the most difficult, as this expands the collapsed lungs by overcoming the high surface fluid tension within. This forces any remaining alveolar fluid into the circulation and drops the high pulmonary artery pressure, leading to establishment of normal cardiopulmonary circulatory flow. If respiratory effort is poor or the infant is centrally cyanosed, continuous positive airway pressure

(CPAP) is helpful both to improve oxygenation and to expand the collapsed alveoli in the lungs. If the child fails to rapidly improve, is apnoic or has a heart rate less than 100/min formal ventilation should be started, and the neonatal crash team alerted. Once the baby is oxygenated, intubation with an uncuffed endotracheal tube should be performed if a skilled operator is available (size 3.5 mm internal diameter (ID) in a term infant, 3.0 mm ID if small-for-dates or preterm. The tube should be no further than 4 cm at the cords to prevent accidental endobronchial intubation). A straight bladed laryngoscope is all that is available usually – this is used to directly lift the epiglottis. Ventilatory rates of 30–40 breaths per minute are used for face mask or endotracheal ventilation.

## Circulation

Neonatal heart rate is best assessed with a stethoscope or by palpating the umbilical cord at its base. If the heart rate is less than 60, or less than 100 with poor respiratory effort or cyanosis, commence external cardiac massage and alert the neonatal crash team. Massage should be performed with the thumbs over the lower half of the sternum and the hands round the chest. The chest should be compressed 2–3 cm, 120–140 times a minute.

Unless there is an underlying cardiac or metabolic abnormality, virtually all neonatal arrests are secondary to hypoxia. Resumption of respiration and restoration of a good cardiac output usually follow rapidly once adequate oxygenation is ensured.

## Intravenous access

In the resuscitation context the umbilical vein is by far the easiest route of access to the neonatal circulation. It can easily be identified in the cord as a large blue superficial structure. If the cord is held taut between the operator's forefinger and thumb an incision can be made in the cord and an umbilical vein catheter passed. A ligature is then applied proximal to the incision. Blood should be taken for blood count, electrolytes, cross-match and sugar. Neonates are prone to hypoglycaemia and this needs careful observation, especially in macrosomic babies. The doses of common resuscitation drugs are shown in Box 4.4.

## Meconium

If meconium-stained liquor is seen during labour, an experienced resuscitator should be present at delivery. If the baby cries

> **Box 4.4** Neonatal resuscitation drugs and fluids
>
> **IV fluid** – Give if capillary refill prolonged or if fetal sepsis or hypovolaemia suspected – colloid or blood 10 ml/kg (suggest: maximum two doses of colloid before considering blood as risk of dilutional anaemia)
>
> **Adrenaline/Epinephrine** – 10 µg/kg endotracheally or intravenously, increase to 100 µg/kg on third dose (IV only)
>
> *Note:  10 µg/kg = 0.1 ml of 1:10 000 (standard Minijet strength)*
> *100 µg/kg = 1 ml of 1:10 000 (standard Minijet strength)*
>
> **Naloxone** – 100 µg/kg intramuscularly. Any child given naloxone for opioid-induced respiratory depression must be admitted to a high dependency observation area as the half-life of naloxone is much shorter than the half-life of most opioids administered in labour, and further respiratory depression may occur
>
> **Defibrillation** – 2 j/kg for the first two shocks, then 4 j/kg
>
> **Ventilation** – Resuscitaires usually have two sources of ventilatory oxygen; a neonatal ambubag with a round face mask, and a pipeline connector with a variable blow-off valve – after connection to the tube occlusion applies a pressure to the valve limit. The valve is usually left at 15–20 cm $H_2O$
>
> **Heat** – Neonates cool rapidly due to evaporative heat loss if damp, high surface to volume ratio and impaired metabolic compensation. They should be vigorously dried as soon as possible after delivery, and then wrapped in warm, dry blankets. The radiant heater on the resuscitaire is designed to keep the baby at a skin temperature of 33–35°C

spontaneously at delivery then it has open airways, and intubation and suction below the cords is not necessary. The baby should be cared for in the normal way immediately post-delivery and no specific action taken to try and suction the airways. If the baby does not cry spontaneously then it should be taken to the resuscitaire and the airway gently cleared of secretions under direct vision. The pharynx should be visualised using a laryngoscope and any meconium seen removed with a suction catheter. It is important to assess the baby's general condition. After initial attempts to clear the airway have been made, the baby should be resuscitated according to the usual guidelines.

**PART II**
# Clinical problems

# CHAPTER 5

# Headache

Headache is a common complaint at any time of life whether pregnant or not, and usually of little consequence. However, it can on occasion be the herald of significant pathology, and thus should always be taken note of. Causes of headache are listed in Box 5.1.

---

**Box 5.1** Causes of headache

**Common**
Tension headache/muscular spasm
Migraine
Drug withdrawal/overuse (prescription or recreational)
Ear, nose and throat (ENT) – sinusitis, otitis
Maxillofacial – temporomandibular joint dysfunction, dental impaction or caries

**Uncommon**
Benign intracranial hypertension
Vascular – subarachnoid haemorrhage, subdural/extradural haematoma, sinus thrombosis
Tumour – benign or malignant
Infection/Inflammation – meningitis, encephalitis, brain abscess
Pre-eclampsia
Carbon monoxide poisoning
Iatrogenic – post-dural puncture (surgical/anaesthetic)

---

The key to assessment of the obstetric patient with headache is to elicit a clear history together with any associated signs or

---

*Handbook of Obstetric High Dependency Care*, 1st edition. By © D. Vaughan, N. Robinson, N. Lucas and S. Arulkumaran. Published 2010 by Blackwell Publishing Ltd

symptoms. A worrying cause can usually be swiftly eliminated, but care should be taken to investigate and treat rapidly those whose presentation is more complex or worrying.

Signs of raised intracranial pressure (Box 5.2) should be sought and, if present, swiftly acted upon. Imaging and neurological referral are vital and guide management.

---

**Box 5.2** Raised intracranial pressure

Signs and symptoms – headache, nausea, vomiting, ocular palsy, decreased level of consciousness, papilloedema
If a mass effect is present causing *displacement of brain tissue*:
Pupil dilation
Sixth cranial nerve palsy
Abnormal respiratory pattern
Cushings triad – hypertension, widened pulse pressure, bradycardia

---

*Tension headache* is the most common cause found. It is often related to physical and emotional stress and usually recurrent. No focal neurology, change in conscious level or other associated abnormalities should be present. Simple analgesia is usually all that is required.

*Migraine* classically presents after prodromal symptoms including scotoma, photophobia and nausea. Patients suffering from migraine are usually familiar with their own symptom set and progression. The headache is usually throbbing and unilateral. Symptoms during an acute attack can be severe (sensory symptoms are common, and aphasia, hemianopia and hemiparesis have been reported) but there are no persistent signs following the attack. Treatment is with analgesics (paracetamol/codeine combinations are safe in pregnancy) and anti-emetics (metoclopramide and cyclizine).

Prophylactic therapy is indicated in those with recurrent episodes. Low dose aspirin is a safe first-line drug. Beta blockade (propanolol) is used in resistant cases though it has been associated with growth restriction in pregnancy. If aspirin fails, specialist input should be sought. The serotonin antagonist pizotifen, whilst very effective outside pregnancy, should only be considered as a last resort as little data exists regarding its safety.

*Drug-related headaches* are seen classically with vasodilators, e.g. glyceryl trinitrate and calcium channel blockers. Prolonged analgesic use and analgesic withdrawal can also precipitate headache.

*Head and neck* related causes are usually chronic. Sinus inflammation is best treated with steroid nasal sprays after specialist review. Antibiotics are rarely indicated and proprietary decongestants, whilst effective initially, often cause a rebound worsening of symptoms in the medium and long term. Dental headache is best referred to a dentist for investigation and treatment, and can be controlled with oral analgesia.

*Benign or idiopathic intracranial hypertension* gives rise to frontal headaches and is a diagnosis of exclusion. It may be associated with papilloedema and diplopia, and is more common in obese patients.

*Intracranial haemorrhage* is classically associated with a sudden and severe occipital headache with associated nausea, vomiting, neck pain, and possible altered consciousness or collapse. Urgent imaging is required (CT/MRI) and referral for neurosurgical review. Intensive care input should be sought early.

*Venous haematoma or thromboses* are most often seen post-partum in the pregnant population. They are associated with signs of raised intracranial pressure and focal neurological signs, though these classically are transient and variable.

*Intracranial infection* (meningitis, encephalitis, abscess) – features include fever, malaise, rigors, photophobia, neck stiffness and nausea. Associated rash, altered level of consciousness and haemodynamic instability are most worrying, and ITU input should be swift. Investigations should be guided by severity and safety of intervention but blood cultures and imaging are mandatory. Antimicrobial therapy should be started prior to confirmation of positive cultures.

*Space-occupying lesions* often present gradually with focal headaches and are associated with worsening localising signs.

*Hypertension/pre-eclampsia* – headache may be severe and associated with other symptoms of pre-eclampsia. A full screen (urinalysis, FBC, clotting, U&Es, creatinine, urate and LFTs) should be sent and measures instituted to smoothly decrease the blood pressure.

## Management

An accurate clinical history is the key to diagnosing the cause of a headache and distinguishing between the various possible causes of headache. Symptoms that should cause particular concern include: sudden onset of headache, increased frequency or severity of headache, headache with underlying systemic illness, focal neurological symptoms (mental state changes or physical symptoms) and headache subsequent to head trauma. A thorough neurological examination must be performed. Clinical findings that mandate neuroimaging are focal neurological signs and papilloedema. Computed tomographic (CT) scanning can be performed with or without contrast and it is essential that requests for CT scanning are accompanied by adequate information so that the appropriate technique is performed. In a patient with a history of sudden onset of headache, neck stiffness and focal neurology, a lumbar puncture should be performed even if the CT scan is normal, as small haemorrhages may not be identified. Cerebrospinal fluid (CSF) analysis (after CT scanning has been performed and excluded raised intracranial pressure) can help to confirm or exclude haemorrhage and infection. Magnetic resonance imaging (MRI) may not be as readily available as CT scanning. However, it has greater sensitivity in detecting brain pathology than CT scanning. The choice of neuroimaging should be made following advice and liaison with the radiology department.

In addition to neuroimaging all patients with suspicious headache should have baseline blood tests for FBC, U&E analysis, liver function tests and serum glucose.

It is mandatory that patients with headaches that are difficult to diagnose, or that worsen or fail to respond to treatment are referred to a neurologist.

## CHAPTER 6

# The collapsed patient

A patient who is found or becomes collapsed on delivery suite is by definition a medical emergency. The causes are many and varied, and whilst obstetric causes are the most likely in an otherwise healthy parturient, it is important not to forget other reasons (Box 6.1).

---

**Box 6.1** Causes of maternal collapse

Shock – Haemorrhage, septic, cardiogenic, uterine inversion
Hypoxia
Embolism
Seizure
Intracranial event
Metabolic

---

Initial treatment is as for any other emergency and as set out in Chapter 3 – ABCDE, oxygen, call for help, basic observations, bloods taken including a sugar estimate and rapid intervention commenced. Immediately, obvious causes of collapse should be treated (convulsion, massive haemorrhage) and rapid attempts made to ascertain the cause. Urgent delivery should be considered as soon as the mother is stabilised to prevent fetal compromise. At times, immediate delivery may be warranted to assist with resuscitation.

Assessment of neurological impairment is best carried out using the Glasgow Coma Score (GCS – see Box 6.2). This not only provides a universally accepted guide to severity but a system to monitor progression with time.

---

*Handbook of Obstetric High Dependency Care*, 1st edition. By © D. Vaughan, N. Robinson, N. Lucas and S. Arulkumaran. Published 2010 by Blackwell Publishing Ltd

**Box 6.2** Glasgow Coma Scale

*Glasgow Coma Scale* or *GCS*, sometimes also known as the *Glasgow Coma Score* is a neurological scale which aims to give a reliable, objective way of recording the conscious state of a person, for initial as well as continuing assessment. A patient is assessed against the criteria of the scale, and the resulting points give a patient score between 3 (indicating deep unconsciousness) and 15 (the more widely used modified or revised scale). The scale was published in 1974 by Graham Teasdale and Bryan J. Jennett, professors of neurosurgery at the University of Glasgow.

The best response in each of the three sections is recorded to derive the final score:

|  | 1 | 2 | 3 | 4 | 5 | 6 |
|---|---|---|---|---|---|---|
| *Eyes* | Not open | To pain | On command | Spontaneously | | |
| *Speech* | None | Sounds | Inappropriate words | Confused | Converses normally | |
| *Motor* | No movement | Extends to pain | Abnormal flexion | Withdrawal from pain | Localises to pain | Obeys commands |

Any score less than 15 is clearly of concern to a clinician but of equal significance is a deteriorating score. A patient with a decreasing GCS needs urgent investigation and treatment.

## Haemorrhage

Obstetric causes include abruption, post-partum haemorrhage, peri-partum trauma and ectopic pregnancy. It may be partially or totally concealed and more likely to be associated with early disseminated intravascular coagulopathy (DIC). Non-obstetric causes are legion but the most common in the obstetric population are trauma, ruptured aneurism and GI bleed.

## Hypoxia

This may be due to a number of causes and is discussed in detail in the following chapters. Severe bronchospasm either pre-existent or secondary to anaphylaxis is the commonest reason in the obstetric population, but upper airway obstruction (oedema, trauma, foreign body), embolus, pulmonary oedema, pneumonia and pneumothorax should all be considered and rapidly treated if present. Ventilatory support (CPAP, formal intubation and mechanical ventilation) may become necessary and should be instituted in the obstetric theatre if necessary until an appropriate HDU or ITU bed is available.

## Embolism

Massive PE presents as collapse associated with central chest pain, sudden onset of breathlessness and signs of right heart strain. Amniotic fluid embolus is seen classically during or after a precipitous delivery. There is increased risk with age, induction of labour, uterine stimulants and hypertonic contractions. Profound shock and haemorrhage due to DIC is seen.

## Seizure (See Chapter 7 for more detail)

Eclampsia may present without warning as a tonic–clonic seizure followed by post-ictal drowsiness. Seizures are best terminated with magnesium sulphate 4 g in a *very slow IV* push. Stabilise the patient and, if antenatal, deliver as soon as is practical. All units will have clear and explicit guidelines as to the management of these patients.

Epilepsy – if no evidence of fetal or maternal compromise and if patient has a history of fits, place in a safe position, give oxygen and wait for seizure to stop. If not stopping or a new presentation, consider magnesium sulphate as above or a short-acting benzodiazepine, e.g. midazolam 5–10 mg in divided IV doses.

## Intracranial event

Subarachnoid haemorrhage will often be preceded with a sudden onset, severe occipital headache and associated nausea, vomiting, neck pain and stiffness and papilloedema. Focal neurological signs are often present. Cerebral infarction most commonly occurs in pregnancy in the post-partum period (first week) and in pre-eclamptic mothers. Ischaemic strokes are usually in the distribution of the carotid and middle cerebral arteries. Those associated with arteriovenous malformations (AVM) tend to occur antenatally however. Sinus thrombosis is usually post-natal, has similar symptoms but of less precipitous onset. Half of patients have gross, transient neurological signs such as hemiparesis.

# Metabolic causes

Hypo- or hyperglycaemia, hypocalcaemia and hyponatraemia can all cause collapse, usually with associated convulsions. A pre-existing diagnosis is usually known (Box 6.3) and treatment is supportive until the cause is established via blood analysis. All collapsed patients should have a bedside blood glucose analysis performed as a matter of course.

---

**Box 6.3** Metabolic causes of maternal collapse

Diabetes
Magnesium therapy
Hyperemesis
Hypoadrenalism
Hypopituitarism
Hypoparathyroidism
Liver failure
Sedative therapeutic or recreational drugs and alcohol

---

# Diabetic crises

These conditions can usually be managed within the obstetric HDU. However, any evidence of persistent haemodynamic instability or reduced consciousness requires liaison with intensive care and may necessitate transfer. *Hypoglycaemia* is rarely encountered in pregnancy unless due to overzealous IV insulin without adequate monitoring. Treatment is supportive with rapid administration of glucose (orally if symptomatic but BM >3, e.g. sugar/Mars bar, IV otherwise or if in doubt – 50 ml 50% dextrose). BM should be regularly measured thereafter as the initial correction may over- or undershoot.

*Hyperglycaemia* is usually asymptomatic. If necessary it can be controlled using a sliding scale of short-acting insulin (Box 6.4). Always ensure that hourly blood glucose monitoring is carried out to adjust the scale appropriately, and that potassium containing fluid is administered concurrently as insulin pushes extracellular potassium into cells, dropping the plasma level. Use 5% dextrose if BM is <12 and saline if over. Regular electrolyte assays should be performed to check sodium and potassium levels.

---

**Box 6.4**  Insulin Sliding Scale Regimen

Use 50 IU Actrapid in 50 ml 0.9% saline. Maintenance fluid should run at 1 l/8 h as a default, with 20–40 mmol K$^+$ added.

| BM (mmol/l) | Infusion rate (ml/h) | Other action |
|---|---|---|
| 0–3.9 | 0 | Recheck in 30 min, give 50 ml; 50% dextrose if <3 mmol |
| 4–7.9 | 1 | |
| 8–11.9 | 2 | |
| 12–15.9 | 4 | |
| 16–19.9 | 8 | |
| ≥20 | 10 | Recalibrate scale upwards. Consult endocrinologist |

---

*Diabetic ketoacidosis* occurs in 1–2% diabetic pregnancies. It is usually associated with a precipitating factor (emesis, infection, poor therapy compliance, steroids and sympathomimetic drugs) and has a high rate of maternal and fetal morbidity and mortality if untreated. Key management features are shown in Box 6.5.

---

**Box 6.5**  Management aims of ketoacidosis in pregnancy

**Fluid replacement**
- 1–2 l of isotonic saline in the first hour
- 300–500 ml/h of 0.9% or 0.45% saline thereafter
- Add 5% dextrose when serum glucose approaches 12 mmol/l

**Insulin therapy**
- Loading dose 0.4 U/kg regular insulin
- Continuous infusion at 6–10 U/h
- Double infusion rate if no response in 1 h
- Decrease infusion to 1–2 U/h as serum glucose drops to 12 mmol/l
- Continue infusion 12–24 h after resolution of ketosis

**Electrolyte replacement**
- Potassium replacement
- Check phosphorus, magnesium

*(Continued)*

**Box 6.5**  (Continued)

**Search for and treat precipitating factor**

*Others*

- Admit to HDU
- Supplemental oxygen
- Place in left lateral position to avoid aortocaval compression
- Monitor fetal HR
- Monitor urine output
- Cause – exclude infection

# CHAPTER 7
# Convulsions

A convulsing patient always causes a huge wave of alarm on delivery suite. There appears to be no control in the situation, the onset is almost always sudden, and relatives and staff alike are prone to panic. It is vital that calm initial management stabilises the situation by ensuring patient safety medically and environmentally, treating the seizure appropriately and then acting swiftly to ameliorate the underlying cause.

The spectrum of neurological disease is vast and complex. However, most patients presenting with a pregnancy and a known neurological condition should present a manageable challenge to the anaesthetist, provided care is taken. Epilepsy is the commonest cause of convulsions during pregnancy, and seizure frequency increases mainly due to subtherapeutic levels of maintenance anticonvulsant therapy caused by altered pharmacokinetics and poor compliance. Antiepileptic drugs may have teratogenic effects on the fetus; so careful preconception advice and follow-up during pregnancy is required from the neurologist. Other causes of seizure should always be remembered (Box 7.1).

Any parturient who has a seizure should initially be managed according to standard core principles. Place them in a safe left lateral position, ABCDE, institute standard monitoring for mother and child (if antenatal) and give supplemental oxygen. Most seizures of whatever cause are self-limiting, and the major management issues are around caring for the post-ictal, drowsy patient, a situation often prolonged if benzodiazepines have been used. Acute control of a convulsion is achieved with magnesium via a slow IV bolus, and/or benzodiazepine administration (midazolam 5 mg plus a further 5 mg if no effect).

---

*Handbook of Obstetric High Dependency Care*, 1st edition. By © D. Vaughan, N. Robinson, N. Lucas and S. Arulkumaran. Published 2010 by Blackwell Publishing Ltd

**Box 7.1**  Causes of seizure during labour

Hypoxia
Hypotension
Epilepsy
Eclampsia
Space occupying intracranial lesion (abscess, tumour)
Cerebrovascular event (intracerebral, subdural or extradural
    haemorrhage; sinus thrombosis)
Drug effects (narcotic overdose or withdrawal, allergy, local
    anaesthetic toxicity)
Metabolic derangement
Sepsis
Amniotic fluid embolus

IV access should be secured and a fluid bolus commenced, baseline observations performed (pulse, pressure, saturation, capillary refill time), and bloods sent for FBC, U&E's, creatinine, glucose, CRP, urate, group and save, liver function tests and clotting. Bedside haemoglobin and glucose estimations should also be performed as well as urinalysis. A full septic screen should be sent if any suspicion exists of infection or sepsis.

If the patient is stable and no further signs are elicited on a full patient examination, note review and seeking other sources of information (midwives, relatives) should clarify any pre-existent cause of fitting. Any evidence of cardiac or respiratory abnormality should be treated swiftly if possible. These are rare but potentially lethal causes of seizure. Senior help (obstetric, anaesthetic and midwifery) should be sought immediately and consideration given to urgent delivery if necessary – the commonest reason for convulsions in pregnancy after epilepsy is eclampsia.

*Eclampsia* is considered to be due to cerebral vasospasm. It is initially managed as above with the primary resuscitation therapy of airway control, left lateral positioning, oxygen therapy, termination of the convulsion and urgent delivery of the fetus if indicated. Further convulsions should be prevented. Specific drug therapy to stop the convulsion includes any of the following: IV diazepam 5–10 mg (which is easily available in the delivery suite), IV thiopentone (which must always be given by an anaesthetist) if in the operating theatre environment or IV magnesium sulphate (Box 7.2)

4 g slowly over up to 5 min (cerebral vasodilator). Magnesium sulphate is indicated after eclampsia to prevent further convulsions for 24–48 h.

---

**Box 7.2**  Magnesium sulphate

**Presentation** – As 50% magnesium sulphate, 10 ml ampoules containing 5 g (20 mmol)
**Dose** – IV bolus followed by infusion, 4 g (40–80 mg/kg) over a minimum of 5 min followed by a maintenance infusion of 1–2 g/h
**Side effects** – Drowsiness, sedation, headache, blurred vision, nausea, constipation, hypotension, cardiac arrhythmias, pulmonary oedema, loss of reflexes, prolongation of neuromuscular blockade
**Overdose management** – Stop drug, supportive treatment, assess blood levels, and consider 10 ml slow IV calcium gluconate or chloride 10%
**Recurrent seizures** – Additional bolus 2 g magnesium sulphate over 5 min with 2 g repeated if necessary 15 min later

---

The clinical and side effects correlate fairly well with the plasma levels of magnesium (Box 7.3).

---

**Box 7.3**  Magnesium: clinical effects and plasma levels

|  | Plasma levels (mmol/l) |
|---|---|
| Normal levels | 0.7–1.0 |
| Therapeutic levels | 2.0–3.5 |
| Widened QRS complex and prolonged PR interval | >3.0 |
| Sedation, severe headache, blurred vision | >4.0 |
| Absent tendon reflexes | >5.0 |
| Heart block, respiratory paralysis, cardiac arrest | 7.5–14.0 |

---

Toxicity can be assessed clinically by measuring the tendon reflexes. If absent the drug infusion regime should be reviewed and blood levels taken. Tendon reflexes in the lower limbs may be decreased or absent if epidural anaesthesia has been given.

If the patient is stable, regains consciousness but no obvious cause is found, further neurological investigation is required, and this is best arranged in consultation with the senior physician or neurologist if available. MRI is widely regarded as the gold standard in imaging for these cases but contrast-enhanced CT is acceptable. It is vital that any patient with convulsions of unknown aetiology be safely monitored and escorted at all times by staff who are able to treat if necessary.

If the fit does not stop or recurs repeatedly, the patient is in status epilepticus (Box 7.4).

---

**Box 7.4** Status epilepticus

**Definition**

A seizure, or series of seizures during which consciousness is not regained, that lasts for at least 30 min

**Management**

This assumes no response to magnesium or benzodiazepines given as above. Senior help should have been summoned and the patient transferred to an appropriate location for monitoring and support. An anaesthetist must be present

If the mother is antenatal and the fetus is of deliverable gestation, rapid sequence induction with thiopentone, intubation and ventilation. Proceed with delivery when stable. Transfer intubated to intensive care. Neuroimaging of brain as soon as possible

If the mother is post-natal or not deliverable, consider phenytoin 20 mg/kg slow IV push (15–20 min). *If unstable proceed as above – intubate, scan, transfer to ITU and discuss with senior neurologist*

---

# CHAPTER 8
# The breathless patient

If a mother becomes ill then recourse to basic principles of care becomes mandatory. The tissues must be oxygenated and for this to occur oxygen must be presented to the lung (via an unobstructed airway). Diffusion of oxygen takes place across the lungs to the blood (carriage being dependant on haemoglobin concentration and adequate red cell mass). The blood containing oxygen is then pumped by the heart to the tissues which utilise the oxygen and excrete carbon dioxide into the blood which diffuses through the lungs and is excreted in breathing.

Assessment of the hypoxic and breathless patient is important and involves both history and examination. Remember that tachypnoea is a good indicator of critical illness from any cause. Once respiratory failure is suspected on clinical grounds, blood gas analysis will confirm and assist in the diagnosis and cause of the mother's illness. Visible cyanosis is a critical sign and is present when the concentration of deoxygenated haemoglobin in the capillaries or tissues is at least 5 g/dl. Confusion, lack of cooperation, hypoxia, myoclonus and seizures can occur with severe hypoxaemia.

## Respiratory changes in pregnancy

Advancing uterine size after the third trimester combined with hormonal changes means that the alveolar minute volume is doubled as pregnancy advances. There is an increased tidal volume and a small increase in respiratory rate at term. This results in the following blood gas analysis for the normal pregnant patient. The partial pressure of $CO_2$ in arterial blood ($PaCO_2$) is reduced by 20% to about 4 kPa (normal non-pregnant state 5 kPa) and the

*Handbook of Obstetric High Dependency Care*, 1st edition. By © D. Vaughan, N. Robinson, N. Lucas and S. Arulkumaran. Published 2010 by Blackwell Publishing Ltd

partial pressure of $O_2$ in the arterial blood ($PaO_2$) is increased by some 10% at term to about 13–14 kPa (normal non-pregnant state 13 kPa). Hypoventilation in the advanced pregnant woman produces cyanosis more quickly than in the normal population for three reasons: (1) oxygen consumption is increased, (2) airway closure of the alveoli may be present and (3) the respiratory reserve (the functional residual capacity) of the patient is reduced. Any pregnant woman who is breathless benefits from sitting upright to minimise these changes and this will improve her oxygenation.

## Differential diagnosis of acute breathlessness – cardiac or respiratory

The causes of breathlessness according to the rate of onset and mechanism are shown in Boxes 8.1 and 8.2.

---

**Box 8.1** Causes of breathlessness according to rate of onset

**Acute (seconds to hours)**
  Pulmonary embolism
  Pneumothorax
  Asthma
  Pulmonary oedema
  Respiratory infection
  Septicaemia
  Cardiac tamponade

**Paroxysmal**
  Pulmonary oedema
  Asthma

**Weeks**
  Cardiac failure
  Recurrent pulmonary oedema
  Pulmonary effusion

---

## Pleuritic chest pain

Pleuritic pain is the most common type of chest pain in respiratory disease and is described as a localised, sharp, stabbing pain aggravated by coughing and inspiration. This pain indicates pleural inflammation, e.g. from infection or embolism and is also a feature of spontaneous

---

**Box 8.2** Common and some rare causes of breathlessness

|  | **Disorder** |
|---|---|
| Airflow obstruction | Asthma |
| Impaired gas exchange | Pneumonia, pulmonary oedema |
| Pleural disease | Pneumothorax, pleural effusion |
| Vascular | Pulmonary embolism |
| Neuromuscular disease | Myasthenia gravis, Guillain–Barre syndrome |
| Extrapulmonary | Obesity, term pregnancy, anaemia |

---

pneumothorax. The causes of chest pain that need to be considered in the differential diagnosis of the patient are shown in Box 8.3.

---

**Box 8.3** Causes of 'sharp' chest pain in the obstetric patient

|  | **Disorder** |
|---|---|
| Pleuritic | Lung inflammation/infection |
|  | Pulmonary embolism |
|  | Pneumothorax |
|  | Rib trauma – fracture |
| Localised muscle pain | Breathlessness and coughing |
| Retrosternal 'raw' pain aggravated by inspiration | Inflamed trachea |
| Costochondral junction pain (2nd ribs bilaterally) | Perichondritis (Tietze's disease) |
| Pain within the region of one dermatome | Herpes zoster |
| Nerve root described as burning | Intervertebral disc |
| Local pain and tenderness of the chest wall muscles | Coxsackie B virus |

---

## Investigations

The cause of the respiratory distress must be found and treatment started. This is paramount but an assessment as to the severity of the illness must also be made. A plan of investigations when combined with appropriate treatment is shown in Box 8.4.

**Box 8.4** Investigations of the respiratory patient

History
Clinical examination
Treatment of specific cause
Medical advice and help
Sputum bacteriology
ECG
Pulse oximetry
Chest X-ray
Blood gas analysis
FBC, U&E, creatinine, blood cultures

After the history and clinical examination there are technical aids to assist with the assessment and management of the patient.

## Oximetry, chest X-ray, arterial blood gases

These are discussed individually in Chapters 10–12. These are important to understand but it is important to reiterate that often the first sign of illness in the breathless obstetric patient is low oxygen saturation as measured by pulse oximetry. Levels under 90% require immediate investigation and treatment with oxygen. The concentration of oxygen given to pregnant patients in the short term can be as much as 100% and do not hesitate to give high percentages of oxygen to ensure tissue oxygen delivery.

Respiratory failure results if gas exchange is impaired and is of two types (Types I or II).

Type I is also called acute hypoxaemic respiratory failure and is the commonest form of respiratory failure. It is associated with all acute lung diseases involving fluid filling or collapse of the alveoli. The hypoxaemia is due to lung ventilation/perfusion (V/Q) mismatch. Hypoxaemia is associated with normal or low carbon dioxide levels.

Type II is ventilatory respiratory failure and results in hypoxia with hypercapnia (raised carbon dioxide). The causes of this are many but can be approached logically. Relevant disorders include:
• Central nervous system respiratory depression – drugs (opioids), intracranial pathology – haemorrhage, stroke, cavernous sinus thrombosis, infection
• Neuromuscular disease – Guillain–Barre syndrome, myasthenia gravis

- Chest wall or pleural disease: pneumothorax, pleural effusion
- Upper airway obstruction: unconscious state, obstruction
- Small airway diseases: asthma

## Treatment principles

The diagnosis and principles of treating the breathless hypoxic patient are shown in Box 8.5. Ask for help. Ensure that appropriate specialists give appropriate advice and that they visit the patient. Consultant care and advice is often needed as junior general doctors are often inexperienced in dealing with sick obstetric patients.

---

**Box 8.5** Treatment principles for improving oxygenation in the hypoxic patient

Differentiate and treat the underlying condition medical, microbiological advice

*If pneumothorax* – chest drain insertion by experienced doctor

*If chest infection* – appropriate antibiotic therapy after consultation with microbiologist, physician and or infectious diseases consultant

*If pulmonary oedema* – diuretic therapy after consultation with cardiologist

*If pulmonary embolism* – further investigations (V/Q lung scan if appropriate) and heparinisation according to local protocols in conjunction with physician's advice

Airway opening manoeuvres

Posture

Analgesia

Physiotherapy

Humidification

Infection control

Oxygen therapy

---

A basic explanation of these principles occurs in the subsequent four chapters and all may be used together to help in the diagnosis and treatment of the respiratory patient.

# CHAPTER 9
# The wheezy mother

Wheeze is a commonly reported symptom. Acute onset of wheeze has many causes and whilst bronchospasm is the most obvious it is important to remember that both infection and pulmonary oedema can present with wheeze. The causes of wheeze are shown in Box 9.1.

---

**Box 9.1** Causes of acute wheeze

Bronchospasm
Asthma
Pulmonary oedema
Pneumothorax
Gastric contents aspiration
Upper airway obstruction
Upper airway secretions
Angioneurotic oedema
Tracheal secretions
Inhaled foreign body

---

## Bronchospasm

Severe bronchospasm or acute asthma needs treatment according to the recommendations below (Box 9.2). It can be life threatening if exhaustion occurs. Signs of exhaustion include:
* Being unable to complete sentences in one breath
* Too breathless to feed

---

*Handbook of Obstetric High Dependency Care*, 1st edition. By © D. Vaughan, N. Robinson, N. Lucas and S. Arulkumaran. Published 2010 by Blackwell Publishing Ltd

- Respiratory rate >25/min
- Pulse rate >125/min, bradycardia, dysrhythmia
- $SaO_2$ <92% despite oxygen therapy
- $PaO_2$ <8 kPa despite oxygen therapy
- $PaCO_2$ >4.5 kPa (hyperventilation normally produces a low normal $CO_2$ and a rising or high $CO_2$ is highly significant of exhaustion)
- Cyanosis
- Silent chest
- Feeble respiratory effort
- Exhaustion
- Coma
- Confusion

The treatment of bronchospasm is shown in Box 9.2.

---

**Box 9.2** Immediate treatment of bronchospasm

High concentration oxygen
Call for help
Intravenous crystalloids – avoid dehydration
Beta 2 agonist via oxygen-driven nebuliser, e.g. salbutamol 5 mg
Consider IV salbutamol if no response
Oral prednisolone 30–60 mg plus or minus IV hydrocortisone
    200 mg
NO SEDATION
Chest X-ray to exclude pneumothorax or consolidation
Consider IV magnesium (2 g infused over 20 min)
Consider IV aminophylline 4–8 mg slowly over 10–20 min (side
    effects include palpitations, dysrhythmia and vomiting)
Consider antibiotics

---

Safe treatment of the wheezy patient is necessary. It is not always easy to clinically detect the difference between wheeze of a respiratory cause from that of a cardiac cause. For example, peri-partum cardiomyopathy can present with a slow onset of cardiac failure which manifests itself as wheeze. Treating this as asthma can delay diagnosis and lead to a potentially fatal outcome.

# CHAPTER 10

# Low oxygen saturation and oxygen therapy

The oxygen dissociation curve is sigmoid shaped and it is important to understand that the oxygen saturation of the patient must be above 90% if tissues are to be adequately perfused. A pulse oximeter is used on the finger commonly and utilises the principle that there is a differing absorption of light at the various (oxygenated and de-oxygenated) states of haemoglobin. Oximetry can be unreliable if there is excessive patient movement, venous congestion or nail polish covering the nails.

Low oxygen saturation (<90%) demands an immediate response and oxygen therapy must be given whilst the cause is sought. Oxygenation of the tissues depends on the following:
- The inspired oxygen concentration
- The lungs: function and diffusion ability
- The haemoglobin concentration
- The cardiac output.

The causes of low oxygen saturation are listed in Box 10.1.

---

**Box 10.1** The causes of low oxygen saturation on pulse oximetry

**Oxygen supply**
Oxygen supply turned on appropriately

**Oxygen delivery**
Tubing and appropriate mask connected to patient
Upper airway obstructed? conscious level satisfactory

*(Continued)*

---

*Handbook of Obstetric High Dependency Care,* 1st edition. By © D. Vaughan, N. Robinson, N. Lucas and S. Arulkumaran. Published 2010 by Blackwell Publishing Ltd

**Box 10.1**  (Continued)

**Lung function normal**
  Bronchospasm?
  Pulmonary oedema?
  Pneumothorax?
  Infection?

**Haemoglobin**
  Haemorrhage?
  Hypovolaemia?

**Heart**
  Adequate blood pressure?
  Arrhythmias?

**Tissues**
  Septicaemia?

The most common cause of low saturation is partial airway obstruction in a semi-conscious patient. Alleviating this problem by a simple jaw thrust will resolve an immediate problem. The other causes need elucidation carefully and systematically.

## Treatment of hypoxia

Support of the respiratory system always involves giving oxygen therapy. Impairment of lung gas exchange causes hypoxia ($PaO_2$ < 10 kPa) with or without hypercapnia (normocapnia is about 5 kPa). The object of treatment is to produce adequate oxygenation and acceptable levels of carbon dioxide excretion.

There are simple measures which can be undertaken to improve oxygenation and a mother's respiratory function. This is independent of the cause of the hypoxia or breathlessness. Whilst making decisions regarding the treatment of a possible pneumonia, pulmonary embolism or possible pneumothorax, the following immediate principles for treatment must be used and these are shown in Box 10.2.

In practice there may be difficulties in identifying and treating the underlying pathology. Empirical treatment may be necessary and it is prudent to ask advice from specialist physicians. Remember the importance of airway opening manoeuvers such as jaw thrust.

> **Box 10.2** Treatment principles for improving oxygenation in the hypoxic patient
>
> Differentiate and treat the underlying condition – medical, microbiological advice
> Airway opening manoeuvres
> Posture
> Analgesia
> Physiotherapy
> Humidification
> Infection control
> Oxygen therapy

Airway obstruction can be subtle and must always be corrected. Attention to posture is important. Sitting the parturient up reduces the weight of the abdominal contents on the diaphragm, increases the functional residual capacity, reduces central blood volume, improves ventilation and reduces left ventricular diastolic pressure. Early mobilisation and sitting out in a chair helps improve the atelectatic lung. Pain after surgery, e.g. caesarean section, inhibits diaphragmatic movement and deep breathing. Physiotherapy is vital. Deep breathing exercises improve lung expansion and helps clear sputum. Humidification with oxygen therapy improves mucociliary clearance and reduces the viscosity of secretions. Remember to be scrupulous about infection control and hand washing as the chances of cross-infection to other patients is always possible.

## Oxygen therapy

Hypoxic patients should be given oxygen therapy. Titrate the inspired concentration (the $FiO_2$) to increase and normalise the patient's oxygen saturation. That means keeping the oxygen saturation above 90%. Oxygen can be delivered to the mother by two different methods – variable performance or fixed performance devices.

### Variable performance devices

These are the face masks and nasal prongs that are commonly seen within the wards and theatres. Examples of this type of mask are the Hudson or MC face mask. These masks draw in a variable amount of air when the patients breathe and are not accurate oxygen delivery devices (they do not provide enough oxygen flow to reach the patient's peak inspiratory flow rate which is 30 l/min). If a patient is breathing normally and the oxygen saturation is being monitored, they deliver a reasonable percentage of oxygen to the patient.

There is 21% oxygen in air. A flow of oxygen of 4 l/min provides about 40% oxygen to the patient and a flow of 6 l/min about 50% oxygen. They are well tolerated by patients and are simple to use and cheap.

Nasal prongs are also well tolerated and do not interfere with eating and drinking but are unreliable as ill patients often breathe through their mouths. Nevertheless, a flow of 2 l/min may provide 40% oxygen to the normally breathing patient.

**Fixed performance devices**

These masks provide an accurate inspired oxygen concentration which is independent of the mother's ventilation (because the flow rate of fresh gas delivered is always higher than the mother's inspiratory flow rate). They work on a high airflow oxygen enrichment (HAFOE) principle. Air is entrained in oxygen to provide concentrations of 24, 28, 35, 40, or 60% oxygen. On the mask the recommended airflow for each oxygen concentration is stated. For example, if 60% oxygen is required to provide adequate oxygen saturation the oxygen flow rate must be set at 15 l/min.

If higher concentrations of oxygen are needed to ensure adequate oxygen saturation, you can use a 'reservoir' mask that uses a collapsible bag into which high flow oxygen is delivered and from which the patient inspires. Valves prevent inspiration from the ambient air and prevent expiration into the reservoir bag. There is always some leak but high concentration approaching 100% oxygen can be delivered this way in an emergency.

If, despite these measures, adequate oxygenation has still not occurred it is possible to apply CPAP to the spontaneously breathing patient. This is achieved by providing special close fitting masks used under anaesthetist supervision. The advantage of CPAP is to keep the alveoli open at the end of expiration which improves oxygenation. The physiology behind this is that the closing capacity of the lung (the total lung volume at which alveoli start to collapse) is within the tidal volume, and CPAP acts to move the range over which tidal movement occurs above this. The disadvantages include hypotension, gastric distension and possible gastric contents aspiration, and it can be uncomfortable and claustrophobic for the patient.

Failure to oxygenate the patient with these measures leads to admission to the ICU and consideration of artificial ventilation.

# CHAPTER 11
# Understanding arterial blood gases

Blood gas analysis assists with both diagnosis and treatment of the sick parturient. An understanding of arterial blood gases is fundamental for safe patient care.

Basically the analysis will display several results. These include the following.

## $PaO_2$ – the partial pressure of oxygen in arterial blood

The normal result for this is about 13 kPa when breathing air in the pregnant population. How this figure arises is as follows. When a patient in health breathes air the atmospheric pressure is 100 kPa (760 mmHg). Approximately one-fifth of air is oxygen and so the partial pressure of oxygen in the air is about 21 kPa (158 mmHg). In the upper respiratory tract there is water saturation of the oxygen and the pressure of it falls to about 19.5 kPa. In the lung alveolus oxygen is taken up by the blood and replaced by excreted carbon dioxide and this reduces the $PaO_2$ in the alveolus to 14 kPa (106 mmHg). As the oxygen diffuses across the lungs to the blood there is always a small gradient or shunt and the arterial $PaO_2$ is always slightly lower than in the alveolus, i.e. about 13 kPa.

When a patient who is healthy breathes 21% oxygen (air) the $PaO_2$ is about 13 kPa and the oxygen saturation is approximately 98%. This patient, when given 40% oxygen will have a $PaO_2$ of about 26 kPa and oxygen saturation still of about 98%. Similarly, when given 60% oxygen the $PaO_2$ will be about 40 kPa and the oxygen saturation will remain at about 99%. A patient who is sick

---

*Handbook of Obstetric High Dependency Care*, 1st edition. By © D. Vaughan, N. Robinson, N. Lucas and S. Arulkumaran. Published 2010 by Blackwell Publishing Ltd

with, pneumonia or asthma, when given 60% oxygen may have an adequate oxygen saturation of 98% but due to 'shunting' of blood through non-ventilated areas of collapsed or infected lung the $PaO_2$ falls dramatically on mixing in the left heart. The $PaO_2$ might be 15 kPa which will provide oxygen saturation to the tissues but is far below that expected in health. This means the patient is very ill.

## $PaCO_2$ – the partial pressure of carbon dioxide in the blood

In the normal population this is 5.3 kPa but as the obstetric population have an increased respiratory rate they 'blow off' carbon dioxide and the normal $PaCO_2$ in the term parturient is about 4.5 kPa. To simplify this, hyperventilation lowers the $PaCO_2$ and hypoventilation elevates it.

## pH – the negative $log_{10}$ of the hydrogen ion concentration

Normal enzyme function in the body depends on a normal concentration of hydrogen ions. The normal pH is 7.35–7.45 and small changes in pH reflect large changes in hydrogen ion concentration as the relation is defined in a logarithmic manner.

### Standard bicarbonate

This standardised value of bicarbonate allows the metabolic component of acid–base equilibrium to be assessed. The normal value is 21–27 mmol/l.

### Actual bicarbonate

This reflects the contribution of both the respiratory and metabolic components and the normal value in venous blood is 21–28 mmol/l.

### Base excess and base deficit

This is a measure of the amount of acid or base that needs to be added to a sample under standard conditions to return the pH to 7.4. It is traditionally reported as base excess and the normal range is +2 mmol/l to −2 mmol/l.

### Oxygen saturation

This in health is about 90% as previously discussed.

## Interpretation of blood gas data

1 Note the clinical picture and the inspired oxygen percentage that the patient is breathing via the mask. Note the $PaO_2$ and the oxygen saturation.
2 Assess the hydrogen ion concentration:
   a pH > 7.45 – alkalaemia
   b pH < 7.35 – acidaemia
   c pH 7.35–7.45 – normal.
3 Assess the metabolic component:
   a $HCO_3$ > 33 mmol/l – metabolic alkalosis
   b $HCO_3$ < 23 mmol/l – metabolic acidosis
4 Assess the respiratory component:
   a $PaCO_2$ > 5.9 kPa – respiratory acidosis
   b $PaCO_2$ < 4.6 kPa – respiratory alkalosis.
5 Combine the above information to determine if there is any respiratory or metabolic compensation.
6 Consider the anion gap which indicates the presence of non-volatile acids (lactic, ketones and exogenous). This is normally 10–18 mmol/l and can be estimated by:

$$(Na + K) - (Cl + HCO_3)$$

Disorders of acid–base balance are divided into acidosis or alkalosis and into those of respiratory or non-respiratory origin. They can be subdivided by the presence or absence of an abnormal anion gap.

## Common disorders of acid–base balance found in the MHDU

### Metabolic acidosis (with a normal anion gap)
Increased gastrointestinal bicarbonate loss, e.g. diarrhoea

### Metabolic acidosis (with an abnormal anion gap)
Lactic acidosis
   Anaerobic metabolism
   Hypotension
   Cardiac arrest
   Sepsis
Ketoacidosis – diabetic

**Metabolic alkalosis**

Loss of acid, e.g. hydrogen loss from the gastrointestinal tract – vomiting, nasogastric suction or hydrogen loss from the kidney – diuretics, hypokalaemia

**Respiratory acidosis**

Respiratory depression – drugs, cerebral injury
Pulmonary insufficiency – pulmonary oedema, pneumonia
Airway obstruction
Muscle weakness – Guillain–Barre syndrome, myasthenia gravis

**Respiratory alkalosis**

Hyperventilation
Hypoxia
Pulmonary embolism
Asthma
Impairment of cerebral function
Early sepsis
Parenchymal pulmonary disorder – oedema

**Mixed disorders**

Metabolic acidosis and respiratory acidosis – cardiac arrest, respiratory failure
Metabolic acidosis and respiratory alkalosis – sepsis and renal failure

Blood gas analysis is not complicated. The most important features are to look for an acidosis. This is serious and often reflects sepsis in the sick patient.

# CHAPTER 12
# The abnormal chest X-ray

At the outset, it is important to state that an acutely sick patient, despite having pathology, may have a normal looking chest X-ray. Often it is several days before pathology such as lung consolidation changes become apparent on an X-ray. Therefore do not assume that there is no pathology if the X-ray is normal – treat the patient, not the picture.

A critically ill patient should not be sent out of the HDU for a chest X-ray. A mobile anteroposterior (AP) film will suffice to assist in the diagnosis of gross pathology.

The plan for interpretation of the chest X-ray is as follows:

## Describe the film

### Date and name
### Orientation
Right/left marker, posteroanterior (PA, radiology department) carries the scapulae shadows laterally, AP (portable ward film). Assume PA unless AP is written on the film.

## Abnormalities

Look for and describe any obvious abnormality first.

### Heart shadow
Normal width is under 50% of the thoracic diameter (PA film) – consider enlarged heart from cardiac failure, cardiomyopathy or mitral valve disease

Abnormal border – consider chamber dilation, overlying lesion

---

*Handbook of Obstetric High Dependency Care*, 1st edition. By © D. Vaughan, N. Robinson, N. Lucas and S. Arulkumaran. Published 2010 by Blackwell Publishing Ltd

Indistinct border – consider lung collapse/consolidation

?calcified valves

## Mediastinum
Hilar enlargement – the left hilum is usually higher than the right by 1–2 cm. The carina overlies T 4/5 on inspiration – consider engorged vascular tree, lymph nodes

## Lungs fields
Equal translucency – consider pneumothorax

Evidence of collapse or consolidation – indistinct heart borders or wedge-shaped appearances, tracheal deviation to the side of the collapse

Pleural effusion – opacification sloping upwards and outwards at the lung base, trachea is pushed away from the midline

Kerley's lines – represent dilatation of the pulmonary vessels as in pulmonary oedema

## Bone structure
Consider rib fractures

## Soft tissues
Position of central venous cannula

Diaphragm – left is usually lower than the right by 2 cm – consider perforated abdominal viscus if air under the diaphragm

Diagnoses in the critically ill mother are difficult. Pulmonary oedema, embolism, pneumothorax, cardiomyopathy and even myocardial infarction are difficult clinical diagnoses in the parturient, and the chest X-ray is often the important test in establishing a firm diagnosis.

# CHAPTER 13
# Chest pain

Chest pain is a symptom which can present with a myriad of others or on its own. It is frequently benign and transient but may herald a catastrophic collapse. It is also one of the greatest causes of worry in the obstetric unit: the possibility of missing a significant event in a patient against the need to devote a considerable period of time and effort to investigate a non-existent pathology.

The key to assessing a parturient with chest pain is rapid and simple intervention combined with accurate history and examination. In the general medical population, chest pain is presumed cardiorespiratory until proven otherwise. This is not a bad concept to hold on to as it reduces the chance of missing serious pathology. Common sense is also necessary – muscular chest wall ache in a patient who has been decorating her house is unlikely to be as serious as sharp central pain and breathlessness in a woman 1 week post-caesarean section. The differential diagnosis of chest pain is shown in Box 13.1.

---

**Box 13.1** Chest pain differential

Gastrointestinal – reflux, peptic ulcer disease
Musculoskeletal – strained muscle, costochondritis, trauma
Respiratory – infection, pulmonary embolus, pneumothorax
Cardiac – angina, infarction, heart failure (though more commonly presents as shortness of breath)
Other – aortic dissection, sickle cell crisis

---

*Reflux* is the commonest cause of chest pain in pregnant women. It is usually burning or sharp, and often postprandial and associated

---

*Handbook of Obstetric High Dependency Care*, 1st edition. By © D. Vaughan, N. Robinson, N. Lucas and S. Arulkumaran. Published 2010 by Blackwell Publishing Ltd

with lying flat. Patients may note regurgitation of food or fluid, and may feel nauseated. There is a rapid response to antacid therapy. No investigation necessary in the absence of other signs. Ask about blood staining in stool or vomit, and consider gastroenterology referral if concerned about possible ulceration.

*Musculoskeletal* pain will be associated with worsening on the use of that muscle group and usually follow a specific event or injury. Chest radiography is not indicated for suspected rib fracture unless severe and thought to be associated with pneumothorax, lung contusion or flail chest – the mechanism of injury usually makes this clear (i.e. bumped on door handle – no; hit by car – yes). Simple analgesics should suffice to treat the pain.

*Respiratory* chest pain is diagnosed from history and examination. Infective causes usually have a sharp pain that is pleuritic in nature. The patient will have associated fever, cough, altered and increased sputum production or be short of breath. Oxygen saturation and blood gas analysis will indicate hypoxaemia in severe cases, and the white cell count and CRP will be raised. Chest radiography may be useful if indicated by clinical findings, and sputum and blood cultures sent. Antibiotic therapy should be based on local guidelines. Admission is mandatory for any hypoxic patient.

*Pneumothorax* presents with acute breathlessness and sharp chest pain. Treatment is by ABCDE, looking particularly for signs of tension (rapid deterioration, deviated trachea, hyper-resonant chest on affected side, altered movement) and consider needle decompression (14G cannula, 2nd intercostal space mid-clavicular line). If the patient is stable and the finding is confirmed on X-ray an underwater sealed drain should be sited.

PE may present as anything from mild, pleuritic pain to crushing central pain to sudden collapse and arrest. This should always be high on the list of possibilities in obstetric patients, and risk is increased in some groups. The onset is usually sudden, associated with severe breathlessness and tachycardia, and sometimes haemoptysis. After resuscitation an ECG may show right heart strain and a chest X-ray should exclude respiratory causes. Arterial gas analysis will show hypoxaemia. Diagnosis is made with a V/Q scan or, more commonly these days, CT pulmonary angiography. Treatment is anticoagulation but this should be discussed with obstetric and medical consultant input urgently sought. This is discussed more fully in Chapter 22.

*Cardiac* causes are fortunately rare in the obstetric population, though increasing in three ways – a small but growing cohort of mothers who have survived congenital heart disease and corrective therapy to maturity but fail to cope with the increased cardiac strain of pregnancy; older mothers with acquired coronary artery disease (smokers, diabetics, family history); and the increasing incidence of valvular heart disease seen largely in immigrant mothers. A classical presentation is of crushing central pain and breathlessness. The pain may radiate to the arm or neck, and is usually precipitated or worsened by increased cardiac work (exercise, labour). Aside from normal supportive/resuscitative measures, diagnosis is clinically supported by ECG changes and elevated troponin and cardiac enzyme levels. Urgent senior cardiological advice and review is mandatory. It should be remembered that neither thrombolysis nor angioplasty are contraindicated in pregnancy if required.

A *sickle cell crisis* should be considered in those with the disease. Those who are Sickle SS or SC will almost invariably know more about their disease than you and be familiar with the signs and symptoms. Analgesia, early CPAP and prompt haematological referral are key.

*Aortic dissection* is rare. It is usually diagnosed when investigating for a possible embolus as the signs and symptoms are similar. Urgent transfer to cardiothoracic surgical care is needed and early, senior anaesthetic involvement vital.

# CHAPTER 14
# Abnormal heart rate, rhythm or ECG findings

Abnormalities of cardiac parameters always cause a degree of anxiety. However, interpretation of these must also consider the physiological state of the patient – a 'normal' HR of 70/min is just as abnormal in a woman in the second stage of labour as a HR of 150/min in a resting antenatal patient. As with all derived signs and investigations, the data they provide are often vital but should never be interpreted in isolation from the patient.

## Heart rate

HR rises during pregnancy as part of the physiological increase in cardiac output. A HR of 100/min is normal at term, and in labour this may rise to over 140/min during contractions and at delivery. Interpretation thus depends on the patient setting. Rhythm is also important and a 12-lead ECG or continuous monitored trace may be useful to assess the electrophysiology. Bradycardia in pregnancy and labour is unusual and should be treated with a high index of suspicion. HR should always be interpreted in association with other parameters (BP, rhythm, oxygen saturation) and other clinical signs or symptoms. Changes related to time are also important; a steadily rising HR with no change in stimulus is a far more worrying sign than one that rises and falls with contractions.

## Heart rhythm

As discussed earlier, relative tachycardia is normal, provided it is sinus. Any other rhythm is by definition abnormal, be it new or

*Handbook of Obstetric High Dependency Care*, 1st edition. By © D. Vaughan, N. Robinson, N. Lucas and S. Arulkumaran. Published 2010 by Blackwell Publishing Ltd

long standing. However, some abnormalities on ECG are accepted as normal variants in pregnancy (Box 14.1).

---

**Box 14.1** Normal variants found on ECG in pregnancy

Relative tachycardia
Increased incidence of both atrial and ventricular ectopics
Left axis shift
Inferolateral T wave inversion
ST depression ($<2\,mm$)

---

## History, examination and investigation

This is clearly helpful in diagnosis of arrhythmia. History taking should include:

- Any history of chest pain or collapse?
- Any shortness of breath on exertion? Ask about exercise and tolerance of exercise. Anyone who can sustain even moderate exercise without undue distress is most unlikely to have a pathological cause.
- Is the patient aware of HR? Is it always fast/slow or just at times? Are there any 'thumps' in the chest, extra or missed beats?
- Is there a history of faintness, dizziness, nausea or chronic fatigue?
- Ask about medication.

### Examination

- Does the patient look well or are there signs of inadequate cardiac output (cold peripheries, peripheral cyanosis or features of congestive cardiac failure)?
- Examination of jugular venous pulse (JVP): elevation in heart failure, cannon waves in complete atrioventricular (A-V) dissociation.
- Careful examination of the pulse and count for at least 30 s.
- Apex shift?

### Investigation

- All usual observations (P, BP, $SaO_2$, urinalysis)
- Bloods – FBC, renal, liver and thyroid function, Ca and Mg, septic screen and CRP

- CTG if antepartum
- ECG and echocardiography if arrhythmia confirmed to exclude structural cardiac causes.

Sinus tachycardia more than 120/min is most commonly due to pain in the peri- or post-partum patient. However, the axiom 'Tachycardia = Hypovolaemia' is a useful one and all inappropriately tachycardic patients should be assumed to be hypovolaemic until proven otherwise. In those who do not have an obvious reason for their fast rate, exclusion of haemorrhage is a first and vital step. This is dealt with fully in Chapter 17.

Non-sinus tachycardia or tachyarrhythmia is pathological, though the mother may be unaware of it. Classification and common symptoms are listed in Boxes 14.2 and 14.3, respectively.

---

**Box 14.2** Classification of tachyarrhythmia

**Supraventricular** – i.e. arising from the conducting system above the A-V node, characterised by narrow QRS complexes on ECG
Atrial flutter
Atrial fibrillation (AF)
Re-entrant tachycardia (often referred to as 'SVT')
Wolff–Parkinson–White (WPW) syndrome

**Ventricular** – arising distal to the A-V node, characterised by broad QRS complexes on ECG
Ventricular tachycardia (VT)
Ventricular fibrillation (VF)

---

**Box 14.3** Common symptoms of tachyarrhythmia

Shortness of breath
Dizziness
Sudden weakness
Palpitations/fluttering in the chest
Light headedness
Syncope/fainting

---

Bradycardia is regarded as a rate below 60/min, though most people will not be symptomatic unless their rate is under 50. It can be caused by a wide variety of pathological processes both intrinsic and extrinsic to the heart. The commonest cause in the obstetric population (who are unlikely to have significant acquired cardiac disease) is drug therapy (Box 14.4), but many other causes should be considered (Box 14.5). Relative bradycardia in a very fit parturient (athlete, professional sportswoman) is acceptable due to vastly superior myocardial conditioning – the authors have seen an Olympian go through labour with no HR above 100/min until delivery, at which point her HR shot up to 160!

---

**Box 14.4** Drug causes of bradycardia

Beta blockers
Calcium channel blockers
Digoxin
Amiodarone
Clonidine
Verapamil

---

**Box 14.5** Causes of bradycardia

Sinus bradycardia
  Physiological
  Drugs (see Box 14.4)
  Endocrine – hypothyroidism, hypoadrenalism
  Neurological – vagal stimulation, Cushing's response, raised
    intracranial pressure
  Hypoxia
  Hypothermia
  Severe jaundice
Sinoatrial block
  Ischaemia
  Hyperkalaemia
  Vagal or other negative chronotropes
Sick sinus syndrome

---

*Reading an ECG* is a subject on which entire books have been written, and is beyond the scope of this book. A brief summary of which parts of the cardiac cycle the various waves and intervals represent is shown in Box 14.6, and a method of reading an ECG is described in Box 14.7.

**Box 14.6**  What the ECG represents

P wave – atrial depolarisation
QRS complex – ventricular depolarisation
T wave – ventricular repolarisation
PR interval – time lag between atrial and ventricular depolarisation
QRS duration – time taken for ventricular muscle to depolarise
QT interval – ventricular depolarisation and repolarisation
R–R interval – duration of ventricular cycle (and thus indicator
   of ventricular rate)
P–P interval – duration of atrial cycle (and thus indicator of
   atrial rate)

---

**Box 14.7**  ECG analysis

**Set-up**
Check patient details (name, date of birth, number), date
   of investigation and any other information recorded –
   symptoms, BP, etc.
Check whether the recording speed and voltage deflection are
   normal (25 mm/s; 1 mV deflection = 1 large square)

**Rates and measurements**
State rate, then the PR, QRS, QT durations
Ascertain the axis

**Rhythm**
State the rhythm. Note any additional features – atrial or ventri-
   cular ectopics
Look for and comment on any conduction block

**Waveforms**
Analyse each in turn – P (?wide/tall/bifid), QRS (?pathological/
   widened/tall), ST segment (?elevated/depressed), T (?inverted/
   large/slurred)

**Diagnosis**
Put it all together. Normal or abnormal? Compare with
   previous if possible. Ask an anaesthetist or cardiologist to
   help if you are unsure

## Management of arrhythmia

Any patient with a symptomatic arrhythmia should have basic resuscitative measures instituted immediately, as stated in Chapter 3. Oxygen therapy, IV access, pulse, BP, oxygen saturation and continuous ECG monitoring are essential. A CTG is advised in any antepartum patient as arrhythmia often leads to a decreased cardiac output and thus may affect placental perfusion. A management sequence is outlined in Box 14.8.

---

**Box 14.8** Initial management algorithm for parturient with arrhythmia

1 Cardiac output present? – palpable pulse, recordable BP. If no, call crash team and commence ALS protocol (see Chapter 4)
2 Cardiac output significantly compromised? – low BP plus symptomatic faintness/altered level of consciousness – urgent intervention required – call crash team/ITU team
3 Cardiac output not significantly compromised – patient aware of symptoms but not distressed/unaware – take precautions as above, investigate and discuss early with anaesthetist and cardiologist

---

Atrial flutter is caused by a re-entrant atrial loop, and typically has an atrial rate of 240–350/min. It is in itself relatively benign but if left untreated may lead to intra-atrial thrombus formation and biventricular dysfunction. Definitive treatment for recurrent episodes is electrophysiological ablation. Acutely it responds well to cardioversion at low energy (20–50 J) but tends to be resistant to chemical therapy, though beta blockers and calcium channel antagonists may be useful to slow the rate.

Atrial Fibrillation is similar to flutter. The serum potassium level should be checked prior to cardioversion (<4mmol/l makes restoration of sinus rhythm less likely) and the patient investigated for precipitating factors (see Box 14.9).

Treatment is usually pharmacological using magnesium, digoxin and/or beta blockade. DC cardioversion may be necessary if the

**Box 14.9** Causes of AF

| | |
|---|---|
| Non-cardiac | Hyperthyroidism |
| | Lifestyle excess – acute usually (alcohol – 'holiday heart', caffeine, cocaine) |
| | Pulmonary embolus |
| | Pneumonia or generalised sepsis |
| Cardiac | Valvular disease (classically mitral stenosis) |
| | Ventricular hypertrophy or cardiomyopathy |
| | Hypertension |
| | Atherosclerotic disease |
| | Sick sinus syndrome |

patient is cardiovascularly unstable. Amiodarone should be avoided if at all possible.

Other supraventricular tachycardias (SVTs) tend to be paroxysmal and recurrent. They usually self-terminate but adenosine is safe to use in the pregnant mother to ascertain the underlying rhythm. If this fails, verapamil or flecainide can be used under cardiological supervision. Cardioversion is rarely necessary.

*Wolff-Parkinson-White (WPW) syndrome* occurs when an accessory conduction pathway exists (the bundle of Kent) which bypasses the A-V node. If an atrial tachycardia occurs the blocking effect of this node doesn't occur and the ventricular rate will match the atrial one. ECG recordings in asymptomatic patients show a shortened PR interval with a slurred upstroke leading to a widened QRS complex. Treatment in an acute arrhythmia is electrical cardioversion, though adenosine can be tried if a defibrillator is also at hand. Other AV node blocking drugs should be avoided as they may worsen the condition. Definitive treatment is by pathway ablation. Any patient with WPW should be discussed with a cardiologist, particularly and urgently if symptomatic.

Ventricular arrhythmias are the most serious and life threatening. VF and pulseless VT are both treated as cardiac arrest. Unstable VT needs urgent cardioversion. The risk of conversion to VF means full operative and resuscitative facilities should be at hand – this should occur in theatre. Stable VT (asymptomatic, uncompromised patient) also carries a risk of deterioration. Medical therapy is the first-line treatment under cardiological supervision (amiodarone, procainamide, sotolol or lidocaine) along with correction of electrolyte abnormalities (particularly low potassium or magnesium). Cardioversion is needed if this fails, though bretylium has been used in refractory cases.

Heart block is usually managed simply with observation unless complete, in which case pacing is required. In acute onset, symptomatic patients this can be via a temporary pacing wire or, if necessary, an external pacer.

## CHAPTER 15
# High blood pressure

Hypertension in pregnancy is the most common reason for admission to the obstetric HDU. We immediately associate hypertension in pregnancy with pre-eclampsia, and for good reason, but other causes should also be considered (Box 15.1). Over 10% of all UK pregnancies are complicated by high blood pressure. About 8–10% of primiparous women will have some evidence of pre-eclampsia, of which 10% (1% of all primips) will have severe pre-eclampsia. Eclampsia occurs in about 0.05% of UK pregnancies, and in 1–2% of pre-eclamptic mothers; 2% of these mothers will die. One of the principle reasons for 2nd and 3rd trimester antenatal care is to detect, treat and protect hypertensive mothers.

---

**Box 15.1** Causes of hypertension in pregnancy

| | |
|---|---|
| Pre-existing | Essential hypertension (diagnosed or new diagnosis) |
| | Rarer secondary causes – renal or cardiac disease, Cushing's or Conn's syndromes, phaeochromocytoma |
| Pregnancy induced | Pre-eclampsia |
| | Pregnancy-induced hypertension (no proteinurea or other pre-eclamptic features) |

---

*Handbook of Obstetric High Dependency Care*, 1st edition. By © D. Vaughan, N. Robinson, N. Lucas and S. Arulkumaran. Published 2010 by Blackwell Publishing Ltd

# Pre-existing hypertension

With our populations increasing maternal age and unhealthy life-style, mothers presenting as diagnosed hypertensives are more common than 20 years ago. New cases diagnosed at booking should be screened for primary causes; no one should be assumed to have essential hypertension. Risks of pre-eclampsia, abruption, premature and small babies are all increased in hypertensive mothers. Those on preconception antihypertensive therapy have a doubled risk of pre-eclampsia.

# Pregnancy-induced hypertension

This usually appears after 20 weeks gestation and resolves within 2 months of delivery. Differentiation between pure hypertension and pre-eclampsia is often difficult, but drug treatment is the same for both (Box 15.2).

---

**Box 15.2** Antihypertensive therapy in obstetrics

| | | |
|---|---|---|
| 1st line | Methyldopa | 250 mg BD to 1 g TDS |
| 2nd line | Nifedipine | 10–40 mg BD (slow release) |
| | Hydralazine | 25 mg TDS to 75 mg QDS |
| | Labetolol | 100 mg BD to 600 mg QDS |
| 3rd line | Doxazocin | 1 mg OD to 8 mg BD |

Post-partum only – angiotensin-converting enzyme (ACE) inhibitors

---

Hypertensive parturients must be followed closely as 20–40% will develop pre-eclampsia, and hypertension may persist post-delivery requiring more long-term drug therapy.

# Pre-eclampsia

The simple definition of pre-eclampsia is the combination of hypertension and proteinurea occurring after the 20th week of a pregnancy. In reality it is a complex multisystem disease caused by vascular endothelial dysfunction. All organ systems may be involved and the disease can present with a multitude of signs and symptoms (Box 15.3).

---

**Box 15.3** Features of pre-eclampsia

**Signs** – Hypertension, proteinurea, oedema, intrauterine growth restriction (IUGR)/death, abruption, maternal convulsions
**Symptoms** – headache, visual anomalies, upper abdominal pain, nausea/vomiting
Investigation results – 24h urinary protein >0.3g, ↑ urate, thrombocytopenia, deranged clotting, deteriorating renal function, haemoconcentration, abnormal LFTs, abnormal umbilical and uterine artery Doppler studies, IUGR, oligohydramnios

---

**Box 15.4** Feto-placental effects of pre-eclampsia

Oligohydramnios
IUGR
Abruption
Death

---

**Box 15.5** Maternal complications of pre-eclampsia

Eclampsia
HELLP syndrome
Pulmonary oedema
Cerebral haemorrhage
Disseminated intravascular coagulopathy (DIC)
Renal failure
Hepatic haemorrhage/rupture

---

The aim of intervention is to prevent the crises related to the disease in the fetus and placenta (Box 15.4) and mother (Box 15.5). Mothers transferred to the obstetric HDU for management of their pre-eclampsia are usually in the more severe stages of the disease. This chapter will focus on their management in the acute setting rather than the general, clinic and community-based antenatal care which is all that most pre-eclamptic mothers require.

# Eclampsia

Any fitting woman who is pregnant (or immediately post-partum) is assumed to be eclamptic until proven otherwise. This is a reasonable assumption but after fit termination a clear diagnosis must be sought (see Chapter 7 for practical management of a fitting woman).

Eclampsia is a grand mal/tonic–clonic convulsion in a patient with features of pre-eclampsia. However, the clinical picture can be confused:

- In up to 20% cases, the presenting symptom of pre-eclampsia is a seizure
- About 80% eclamptic fits are in obstetric units
- Fitting is common post-partum (antenatal 38%, peri-partum 18%, post-partum 44%)
- Risk decreases with increasing age

# Management of uncontrolled hypertension

Therapeutic options are shown above for control (Box 15.2). Failure of therapy necessitates rapid intervention. Each unit will have a protocol for this, but the principles are as follows:

- Transfer to HDU.
- Ensure normovolaemia (pre-eclamptics are often intravascularly depleted). Consider central venous access for monitoring. Post-partum, oliguria is normal in mothers; don't be overzealous in chasing a urine output. Aim for 1 l every 12 h input to start, and accurately record input/output.
- Hypertensive control is vital, but it must be remembered that this only controls the symptom, and does not treat the disease process. Consider labetolol, hydralazine or nifedipine according to protocol. Systolic pressures over 160 mmHg are associated with cerebrovascular accident and must be treated.
- The treatment of pre-eclampsia is delivery. Control of pressure is important but should not override a clinical indication to deliver. Strong indications for urgent delivery are uncontrollable blood pressure, compromised fetal condition, deteriorating liver or renal function and deranged clotting.

*Post-partum antihypertensive treatment* depends on severity and duration of hypertension. For those with pre-existing hypertension it is normal to return them to their usual therapy. The options for the persistently new post-partum hypertensives are summarised in Box 15.6.

**Box 15.6** Post-partum antihypertensive treatment

Stop methyldopa (increases risk of post-partum depression).
Add in drugs as needed in the order given or according to local
protocol.

1  Beta blocker (atenolol 50–100 mg OD)
2  Calcium antagonist (nifedipine 10–20 mg BD) OR ACE
   inhibitor (enalapril 5–10 mg BD)
3  Labetolol (alpha and beta blockade)
4  The other drug not used from Point 2

All the above are safe for breastfeeding. Post-partum hypertension usually settles by 6–8 weeks. Anyone still requiring
therapy at this time should be referred to cardiology/their GP
for long-term follow-up.

# CHAPTER 16
# Low blood pressure

Hypotension has a myriad of causes in parturients, but the key diagnosis is to exclude haemorrhage. Other causes are more common or may be more serious, but the levels of morbidity and mortality associated with perinatal haemorrhage (particularly if not treated aggressively and promptly) make its early exclusion from the diagnostic process vital.

The principal causes of hypotension in parturients are listed in Box 16.1.

---

**Box 16.1** Common causes of hypotension

*Shock* – haemorrhagic, cardiogenic, septic, anaphylactic, obstructive (embolus), neurogenic, trauma

*Obstetric* – uterine rupture/inversion, genital tract trauma, uterine hypotonus, cord prolapse, precipitous labour and cervical stretch

*Cardiovascular/Circulatory* – arrhythmia, pump failure (infarction, cardiomyopathy and tamponade)

*Respiratory* – pneumothorax (particularly tension), pneumonia, severe bronchospasm

*Abdominal* – hepatic or renal failure, pancreatitis, intra-abdominal infection/infarction/obstruction

*Endocrine* – hypoglycaemia, Addison's disease, hypothyroidism

*Drugs* – antihypertensive therapy, tocolytics, oxytocics

*Iatrogenic* – regional anaesthesia (can occur with correctly placed epidurals but beware 'total spinal' – high block from inadvertent intrathecal injection of local)

---

*Handbook of Obstetric High Dependency Care*, 1st edition. By © D. Vaughan, N. Robinson, N. Lucas and S. Arulkumaran. Published 2010 by Blackwell Publishing Ltd

# Management of hypotension

The initial management of hypotension is aimed at the simultaneous correction of the low BP to preserve maternal oxygen delivery, and the diagnosis of the cause to prevent recurrence. The principles outlined in Chapter 3 are used, and for this case these are summarised in Box 16.2.

---

**Box 16.2**  Initial management of hypotension

*A – Airway* – clear airway, apply high flow oxygen via a rebreathing mask, lie patient down with a tilt or wedge if antepartum, call for help (senior obstetrician, anaesthetist and midwives) and ask midwife to attach monitoring (P, BP, saturation and CTG)

*B – Breathing* – rapidly assess – look, listen and feel. Treat tension pneumothorax if suspected

*C – Circulation* – assess pulse (rate, rhythm, fullness). Recheck BP. Establish any obvious source of haemorrhage. Site 2 large IV cannulae (16 g at least) and draw blood at the same time for FBC, clotting, cross-match, U&Es, LFTs, urate, CRP. Start fast IV infusion (Hartmans 1L each line).

If there is obvious haemorrhage, instruct someone to call switchboard and put out a major haemorrhage alert to free more staff and resources. Consider using O negative blood if haemorrhage is torrential.

If a cardiac cause is suspected check monitor and request an urgent 12-lead ECG.

*D – Disability* – briefly assess conscious state (AVPU)

*E – Exposure* – full assessment including abdominal and vaginal (concealed bleed, uterine rupture, etc.)

---

The management of haemorrhage (Chapter 17) and the other major causes of hypotension are discussed elsewhere within this section. The remainder of this chapter will thus cover those rarer causes not mentioned elsewhere – obstetric, anaesthetic, drug and endocrine causes.

## Obstetric emergencies

*Uterine rupture* occurs in approximately 1:10 000 pregnancies. One-thirds of these are antenatal (almost exclusively 3rd trimester) and the rest during labour. The causes are listed in Box 16.3.

---

**Box 16.3** Causes of uterine rupture

**Antenatal**
*Trauma*
*Spontaneous* (particularly if polyhydramnios, big or multiple fetus)

**Perinatal**
*Spontaneous* in high risk patients with previous uterine surgery (particularly classical caesarean section or myotomy for fibroid removal), abnormal uterine anatomy (e.g. underdeveloped uterine horn)
*Iatrogenic* – oxytocics, instrumental delivery, internal version

---

The diagnosis may be unclear so the treatment is simple, combined urgent surgical delivery and resuscitation.

*Uterine hypotonia* is treated initially with massage, compression and uterotonic drugs (oxytocin, ergotamine and prostaglandins). Further measures include an intraluminal balloon, brace suture and, in extremis, hysterectomy. Recent advances in radiological embolisation techniques have reduced the need for the latter. Always ensure a full vaginal examination has excluded haemorrhage from the cervix, vagina or perineum.

*Uterine inversion* is very rare (~1:10 000 deliveries) but is fatal in up to 15% cases, hence prompt treatment is vital. Tocolytics may be of use but urgent general anaesthesia for relaxation and manual or surgical correction are the only reliable treatment.

## Anaesthetic causes

The most common anaesthetic cause is *hypotension after routine epidural/spinal* for labour. Ensure that there is no aortocaval compression (move patient onto her side or use a wedge) and apply at least 40% oxygen. If there is no response to an initial fluid bolus of 300–500 ml, give ephedrine 3–6 mg, titrated to effect. Do not use an α-agonist as these agents worsen already compromised placental perfusion.

*'Massive' spinal* – occurs when an epidural dose of local anaesthetic is given into the CSF due to inadvertent and unrecognised catheter misplacement. Clinically there is a rapid ascent of block associated with hypotension and, if the mixture reaches the brainstem, apnoea. Summon help as soon as the diagnosis is suspected. Treatment is supportive – ventilation, IV fluids and ephedrine as required. Continuous fetal monitoring is mandatory and a low threshold should exist for urgent caesarean section to deliver the baby.

## Drug causes

*Antihypertensive therapy* is usually well tolerated by parturients. The exception to this can be in the acute management of uncontrolled pregnancy-induced hypertension, when bolus doses of IV labetolol or hydralazine are used. These can produce rapid and profound drops in BP, and for this reason should be given in the HDU environment whilst the mother is closely monitored.

*Tocolytics* are β-adrenoceptor agonists and thus may cause hypotension via a vasodilatory response.

*Oxytocin* and *ergotamine* both may cause either hyper- or hypotension. Monitoring after dose administration is mandatory.

## Central venous access and pressure measurement

Central venous access is used for a variety of reasons (Box 16.4). A sterile catheter, often multilumen, is placed in the subclavian or

---

**Box 16.4** Indications for central venous access

Fluid resuscitation
Measurement of CVP
Parenteral nutrition
Administration of irritant drugs
Difficult peripheral venous access

internal jugular vein under aseptic conditions. This type of IV access has many advantages over standard peripheral access, but these must be balanced against the risk of complications (Box 16.5).

---

**Box 16.5** Complications of central venous access

*Immediate* – failure, malposition, arterial puncture, pneumothorax, arrhythmia, haemorrhage
*Early and late* – air embolus and haemorrhage (disconnection)
*Late* – infection/sepsis, haemorrhage from internal vessel erosion

---

CVP measurement can be performed once a line has been sited and confirmed both clinically and radiologically to be correctly sited. CVP is the pressure in the right atrium of the heart. This can be used to assess the filling status of the CVS in situations where this is unclear (major haemorrhage) or where there is concern that excessive fluid filling may cause failure and pulmonary oedema (severe pre-eclampsia, pre-existent heart failure). It is important not to use individual readings but to look at the trend over time and response to fluid bolus doses – minimal rise indicates under filling, a rise and slower fall is a normovolaemic response and a rise with no fall indicates the mother is overfilled.

# CHAPTER 17
# Bleeding and transfusion

There has been an impressive decline in the number of deaths from obstetric haemorrhage over the 20 years. However, worldwide it remains a leading cause of maternal death, accounting for 30% of maternal deaths. Although data surrounding maternal morbidity is less comprehensive than for mortality, haemorrhage has been shown to account for two-thirds of all cases of maternal death in two major surveys. Furthermore, the Scottish study on maternal morbidity showed that this rate is not declining (Box 17.1). Haemorrhage is the most common reason for admission to a MHDU.

| **Box 17.1** Scottish maternal morbidity study | | | |
|---|---|---|---|
| **Year** | **Total number of women** | **Number of severe haemorrhages** | **Percentage of total admissions** |
| 2003 | 270 | 176 | 65 |
| 2004 | 246 | 171 | 69 |
| 2005 | 329 | 235 | 71 |

Significant advances have been made in the management of obstetric haemorrhage over the last decade.

## Cause and risk factors of obstetric haemorrhage

Risk factors that are commonly listed as putting a woman at risk of obstetric haemorrhage are multiparity, multiple pregnancy

*Handbook of Obstetric High Dependency Care*, 1st edition. By © D. Vaughan, N. Robinson, N. Lucas and S. Arulkumaran. Published 2010 by Blackwell Publishing Ltd

and previous caesarean section. The demographics of the obstetric population in the UK have changed in the last 10 years and there are 'new' factors that should also be considered (Box 17.2).

---

**Box 17.2** Risk factors for obstetric haemorrhage

**'Traditional'**
• Multiple pregnancy, polyhydramnios
• Previous caesarean section/myomectomy
• Multiparity

**'New'**
• Obesity
• Older mums
• Large babies > 4 kg
• Unbooked parturient
• Ethnicity
• Rising caesarean section rate

---

It is unclear why woman from ethnic minorities are more at risk of obstetric haemorrhage, but is likely to be related more to social issues and reduced access to appropriate healthcare.

Traditionally the causes of obstetric haemorrhage have been divided into antepartum and post-partum but perhaps a more useful functional classification is that of the 'four Ts' (Box 17.3).

---

**Box 17.3** The four 'T's of obstetric haemorrhage

| Four Ts | Cause | Approximate incidence (%) |
|---------|-------|----------------------------|
| Tone | Atonic uterus | 70 |
| Trauma | Lacerations, haematomas, inversion, rupture | 20 |
| Tissue | Retained tissue, invasive placenta | 9 |
| Thrombin | Coagulopathies | 1 |

# Management of obstetric haemorrhage

A patient should only be admitted to the obstetric HDU after the haemorrhage has been stopped. The underlying principles of management of the patient with obstetric haemorrhage also dictate ongoing care on the MHDU. These are:

*   Recognition and resuscitation
*   Teamwork
*   Stop bleeding
*   Aftercare.

## Recognition and resuscitation

Uterine blood flow is 700 ml/min at term and obstetric haemorrhage can rapidly become torrential. However in general, pregnant women are healthy and this combined with the physiological changes of pregnancy mean that they are able to tolerate blood loss well. They will maintain a normal HR and BP until blood loss becomes critical. It has been estimated that blood loss may reach 40% before signs of shock become apparent (Box 17.4). In addition disseminated intravascular coagulation may develop rapidly in the obstetric patient because of placental abruption, amniotic fluid embolus or intrauterine fetal death. A further important consideration is that blood loss in the obstetric patients may be concealed. Therefore to rely on monitoring pulse and BP alone, as indicators of hypovolaemia is inadequate and may lead to either complete failure of recognition of ongoing haemorrhage or failure to recognise the extent of blood loss. This has been a consistent finding in the Confidential Enquiry reports. Of equal importance when assessing an obstetric patient for blood loss is assessment of end organ perfusion, in particular

---

**Box 17.4** Key components of assessment of obstetric haemorrhage

*   HR and BP
*   Fetal assessment, e.g. CTG in antepartum patient
*   Urine output
*   Regular assessment of haemoglobin concentration
*   Assessment of lochia
*   Fundal height in post-partum woman

the kidneys. In haemorrhage, HR and BP will be maintained at the expense of kidney perfusion and the assessment of urine output is as important as monitoring the CVS. Another extremely useful and sensitive indicator of haemorrhage is the bedside assessment of haemoglobin with the hemocue® device. Even in the best units there will be a turnaround time for laboratory haemoglobin levels. The hemocue provides a rapid and accurate assessment of a patient's haemoglobin. More recently introduced onto the market are bedside co-oximeters which can provide a continuous assessment of a patient's haemoglobin. Lastly as haemorrhage may be concealed in a woman who has delivered, regular assessment of the fundal height of a patient's uterus is essential.

## Resuscitation

Resuscitation of the patient who has suffered obstetric haemorrhage follows the principles of resuscitation of all patients, ABC. Volume resuscitation of the patient who has suffered obstetric haemorrhage has two components:

1 *Adequate intravenous access.* Intravenous access in this situation mandates two large bore cannulae (14G or 16G, grey or brown). It may be necessary to site an arterial line and CVP line but these are not needed in the acute situation.

2 *Adequate volumes of fluid.* A discussion on the relative merits of crystalloids and colloids is outside the scope of this book. Systematic reviews reveal uncertainty about the best way to restore circulating volume in hypovolaemic shock. There is no firm evidence that the use of any colloid solution is superior or associated with better patient outcomes than crystalloids. Some colloid solutions affect haemostatic function and so could contribute to a bleeding tendency.

Crystalloids and colloids can restore normovolaemia initially but it is essential that blood transfusion is not delayed in obstetric haemorrhage. If cross-matched blood is not available it is acceptable to use group specific or group O Rhesus negative blood whilst waiting. It is essential that fluids and in particular cold blood are infused through a warming device.

## Coagulopathy

Obstetric haemorrhage may be associated with the development of significant coagulopathy either as a result of clotting factor/platelet count dilution by infusion of large volumes of crystalloids/colloids/

packed red cells or by the development of disseminated intravascular coagulopathy (DIC). DIC results from activation of the coagulation and fibrinolytic systems leading to consumption of platelets, coagulation proteins, fibrinogen and platelets. Ideally transfusion of all types of blood products should be managed with evidence from laboratory investigations; however in obstetric haemorrhage because of the rapidity and severity with which it can develop it is likely to be necessary to give products (particularly coagulation support) on clinical grounds only.

## Risks and complications of blood transfusions

The risks and complications of blood transfusion may be classified as early and late (Box 17.5).

The UK blood transfusion and tissue transplantation services have produced an excellent 'Handbook of Transfusion Medicine' easily accessible on the internet (http://transfusionguidelines. org/docs/pdfs/htm_edition-4_all-pages.pdf) with comprehensive guidance on the management of any suspected transfusion reaction.

---

**Box 17.5** Risks and complications of blood transfusion

**Early**
- Incorrect blood transfusion due to clerical error in the laboratory or at the bedside leading to acute haemolytic transfusion reaction
- Reaction due to infected blood
- Allergic reaction/anaphylaxis
- Febrile non-haemolytic transfusion reactions
- Hypothermia
- Electrolyte disturbance – hyperkalaemia, hypocalcaemia, acid–base disturbance
- Circulatory overloads
- Air embolism
- Transfusion-related acute lung injury

**Late**
- Transfusion of disease
- Delayed haemolytic transfusion reaction
- Post-transfusion purpura

## Teamwork

Communication and good teamwork are an essential part of the management of obstetric haemorrhage. A consistent recommendation in Confidential Enquiry reports is that all hospitals must have locally agreed protocols for the management of obstetric haemorrhage with regular practice 'fire drills'. Most hospitals now employ a 'massive obstetric haemorrhage call' to activate the multidisciplinary team and processes required to manage obstetric haemorrhage safely (Box 17.6).

---

**Box 17.6** Key components of massive obstetric haemorrhage call

Call to switchboard to summon help from senior obstetrician and anaesthetist
Alert haematology laboratory – transfusion and request urgent cross-matched blood
Alert consultant haematologist
Alert portering services for transport of blood products/blood samples

---

Fire drills are dummy clinical scenarios of obstetric emergencies. All staff should take part in these rehearsals of procedures and protocols to ensure as far as possible that in the real event successful management occurs.

## Cell salvage

Concerns about the risks and complications associated with allogeneic blood have led to renewed interest in the use of cell salvage in obstetrics. Cell salvage has not been routinely employed in obstetrics because of safety concerns regarding embolism, or haemolytic disease as a result of re-infusion of fetal cells or amniotic fluid.

During intra-operative blood cell salvage during caesarean section, blood that is lost during the operation is aspirated from the surgical field using a catheter. The blood is then suctioned in a reservoir in which a filter removes gross debris. The filtered blood is then washed and re-suspended in saline for transfusion, which may be re-transfused either during or after the operation.

A leukocyte depletion filter may also be used in this process to reduce the number of leukocytes in transfused blood which may reduce adverse reactions to re-infused blood and limit disease transmission.

A recent major review of cell salvage in obstetrics (Allam, 2008) concluded that autotransfusion following cell salvage in obstetrics does not appear to increase the rate of amniotic fluid embolism, infection or disseminated intravascular coagulation. Its use in unexpected major haemorrhage or in cases at increased risk of major haemorrhage was recommended. It may not be practical to use in the MHDU itself but should be considered in patients who require surgical intervention to manage haemorrhage.

### Stopping the bleeding

Early identification of the cause of haemorrhage is essential to a good outcome. Obstetric haemorrhage can rapidly become torrential with all the concomitant problems of massive haemorrhage and transfusion. Treatment depends on the cause and can be classified as physical, pharmacological, surgical and radiological (Box 17.7).

---

**Box 17.7**  Management of obstetric haemorrhage

**Physical**
- Rubbing up uterine contractions
- Warm packs

**Pharmacological – oxytocics**
- Syntometrine: syntocinon 5 units with ergometrine 500 mcg intramuscular (IM) injection
- Syntocinon: 5 units, slow IV bolus, may be repeated once if necessary, followed by 40 units/500 ml infusion over four hours
- Ergometrine: 0.5 mg IM injection
- Carboprost: (Hemabate or prostaglandin F2a) 250 mcg IM (not IV) may be repeated every 15 min to a maximum of 8 doses
- Misoprostol 400–800 mcg – PR

**Surgical treatment**
- Removal of retained products
- B lynch suture
- Uterine tamponade with Rusch balloon
- Hysterectomy

**Radiological**
- Uterine arterial embolisation or balloon occlusion

---

The pharmacological treatments of obstetric haemorrhage can themselves cause complications which have to be managed on the MHDU. These are summarised in Box 17.8.

---

**Box 17.8** Side effects of pharmacological treatments of obstetric haemorrhage

| Drug | Side effects |
|---|---|
| Syntocinon | Hypotension and tachycardia<br>Antidiuretic effect leading to reduced urine output and hyponatraemia |
| Ergometrine | Hypertension (therefore contraindicated in pre-eclampsia/eclampsia)<br>Vomiting |
| Misoprostol | Nausea, vomiting, diarrhoea, abdominal pain, rashes and dizziness |
| Carboprost | Bronchospasm, pulmonary oedema |

---

### Women who decline blood transfusion

The majority of women will accept blood products if the clinical reasons for their use are fully explained. However, a few may decline blood products because of personal or religious beliefs, e.g. Jehovah's Witnesses.

Ideally these women should be noted well in advance of delivery so that a management strategy for the prevention and treatment of haemorrhage can be prepared. This strategy should include general measures such as optimisation of haemoglobin levels pre-delivery with erythropoietin and iron, the use of oxytocics at delivery and timely attention to the repair of perinea trauma. The threshold for medical intervention at the first sign of obstetric haemorrhage should be lower than for other patients.

Documentary evidence, e.g. a checklist, detailing blood products that will be accepted in the event of massive obstetric haemorrhage (see below) should be completed, signed and witnessed and a copy placed in the medical record and its contents respected.

# CHAPTER 18

# Rashes and itching

The onset of a rash to a patient in the HDU can be highly significant. There are three main causes of acute rashes that need differentiation and treatment. These are:
- Drug reactions
- Infections
- Other disorders.

## Urticarial disorders

Urticaria (hives) describes the itchy, erythematous weals that arise acutely from mast cell degranulation. These commonly arise after *drug reactions* in this environment. The precipitating drugs are most likely to be antibiotics, opiates and non-steroidal anti-inflammatory drugs (NSAIDs). Stopping the drug stops the itching and swelling, which is often confined to the hands and feet, within minutes to hours. Occasionally when the causative drug is administered angio-oedema and, rarely, anaphylaxis may occur. The patient may collapse and rarely cardiac arrest can be precipitated. Epinephrine is indicated and this is discussed in Chapter 26. It is important to remember that cutaneous drug allergy can manifest itself up to 3 weeks after the causative drug has been given.

The complaint of pruritis is not uncommon in pregnant women. Itchiness without either a rash or any evidence of cholestasis can occur in up to 20% of pregnancies. Any pregnant woman complaining of itch without a rash needs LFTs to exclude a hepatic cause (Chapters 20 and 25).

The basic causes of itching are shown in Box 18.1.

*Handbook of Obstetric High Dependency Care*, 1st edition. By © D. Vaughan, N. Robinson, N. Lucas and S. Arulkumaran. Published 2010 by Blackwell Publishing Ltd

---

**Box 18.1** Causes of itching

Physiological
Drug reactions
Liver disease
Primary skin diseases

---

## Infections

Most, but not all, skin infections are due to gram positive cocci. The most important question to be addressed, once a drug-induced urticarial disorder has been excluded, is whether or not the patient is systemically ill. If there is evidence of generalised sepsis (tachycardia, tachypnoea, hypotension, oliguria and pain) and a rash, the diagnosis of *necrotising fasciitis* must be considered. Delay in this diagnosis can be fatal for the patient. These patients need acute surgical debridement, and medical help must be sought to ensure correct antibiotics are given and the patient must be transferred to the ITU. If there is a rash in which there is tenderness, swelling and an ill-defined erythema around a wound, or in an oedematous leg in a patient who is well (only pyrexia), *cellulitis* of the subcutaneous tissue is the most likely diagnosis. Cellulitis and impetigo are normally caused by staphylococci and erysipelas by streptococci. Skin infections are not easy to diagnose and advice from the on-call dermatologist must be sought. Microbiological advice must be sought when prescribing antibiotics.

## Other disorders

Other rashes are not likely to need such acute treatment and dermatological advice, which is often readily available, must be sought. The dermatoses specific to pregnancy that present in the peri-partum period are polymorphic eruption of pregnancy, pemphigoid gestationis (serious, and patients may be on immunosuppressives), pruritis of pregnancy and pruritic folliculis of pregnancy. These diseases, in general, are rare, but may present at term and usually self-resolve after delivery.

# CHAPTER 19
# Temperature and infection

Normal body temperature is maintained at between 36°C and 37.5°C and normal metabolic function of the body occurs at temperatures within this range. There are no alterations within this range of normality in pregnancy and the peri-partum period. All changes in temperature are, therefore, significant.

## Hyperthermia or pyrexia

Hyperthermia or pyrexia is defined as a temperature >37.5°C. Pyrexia increases the metabolic rate and oxygen consumption which precipitates an increase in cardiac output and minute ventilation to meet this demand. The pregnant woman has less reserve than normal as these changes are part of her normal physiology. The higher metabolic rate results in increased carbon dioxide production and this is initially compensated for by further tachypnoea. However, as the patient tires she may develop a respiratory acidosis. This is further compounded by a metabolic acidosis which is caused by an increasing oxygen debt and lactic acidosis. Sweating and vasodilatation cause hypovolaemia which exacerbates the maternal condition. If this situation is left untreated CNS dysfunction (delirium, seizures, coma), rhabdomyolysis, acute renal failure (ARF), myocardial ischaemia and death may follow.

The causes of pyrexia are shown in Box 19.1.

General cooling measures should be adopted. Exposing the patient to cool air fans is beneficial as is prescribing antipyrexial drugs such as paracetamol but it is most important to identify and treat the cause.

*Handbook of Obstetric High Dependency Care*, 1st edition. By © D. Vaughan, N. Robinson, N. Lucas and S. Arulkumaran. Published 2010 by Blackwell Publishing Ltd

> **Box 19.1** Causes of pyrexia
>
> Sepsis
> - Endometritis
> - Urinary tract
> - Episiotomy
> - Abdominal incision
> - Lung infection
> - Breast
> - Legs – phlebitis
> - Epidural site
> - Systemic concomitant disease – e.g. influenza
>
> Blood transfusion reactions
> Environmental – warm fluids, warming blankets
> Drugs – atropine overdose, drug interactions, neuroleptics
> Endocrine – hyperthyroidism, phaeochromocytoma
> Hypothalamic injury – cerebral hypoxia or oedema

## Hypothermia

Hypothermia is defined as a core temperature <35°C. This is normally an accidental occurrence in this environment. It can arise intra- and post-operatively from the causes shown in Box 19.2.

> **Box 19.2** Factors predisposing to post-operative hypothermia
>
> Ambient theatre temperature
> Young mothers
> Surgery – duration
> Concomitant disease
> Cold IV fluid administration
> Drug therapy – vasodilators such as hydralazine and labetolol

Prevention of heat loss can be undertaken by the correction of any ambient temperature abnormality, airway humidification, skin warming measures (passive insulation of the patient or active warming by a forced hot air warmer) and warm IV fluids.

## Sepsis

Doctors must be clear about definitions in sepsis. The systemic inflammatory response syndrome (SIRS) is tachycardia, tachypnoea, pyrexia or hypothermia, or a WBC >12 000 mm$^3$ or <4000 mm$^3$ whilst sepsis is SIRS + a confirmed infectious process. The Sepsis Syndrome (severe sepsis) is SIRS + a confirmed infectious process + organ dysfunction.

It is imperative in any unstable patient to consider sepsis within the differential diagnosis. Early symptoms and signs are usually non-specific (tachypnoea can be an early significant sign) and it is not uncommon for a routine blood test abnormality (white cell count, rising CRP) to be found which will alert the medical staff to occult sepsis.

A patient can have dual pathologies, i.e. two obstetric conditions at the same time, and it is important to remember this. If a patient has severe pre-eclampsia she may have symptoms relating to this primary disease but may also have sepsis. The signs of pre-eclampsia can cloud and compound the symptoms, signs and investigations of sepsis.

Most infections of obstetric origin are polymicrobial involving aerobic and anaerobic organisms indigenous to the genital tract and commonly include streptococci, *E. coli, Klebsiella* and bacteroides species. Predisposing factors for puerperal sepsis include:
- Caesarean section
- Prolonged labour and membranes rupture
- Traumatic vaginal delivery
  - Forceps
  - Episiotomy
  - Retained placenta
  - Repeated vaginal examinations
  - Intrauterine manipulation
- Low socio-economic groups

The first assessment is a *clinical* review of the patient: a detailed history and a full examination are necessary. Normally puerperal sepsis presents with a temperature, lower abdominal pain and uterine tenderness. Untreated it will lead onto malaise, anorexia, foul lochia and severe abdominal pain. A pelvic abscess may develop when a spiking temperature, vomiting, lower abdominal pain, ileus and a tender abdominal mass may be palpated in the pelvis. In the general examination, two phases of sepsis may be distinguished.

1 Hyperdynamic phase – warm pink patient with bounding pulse
2 Hypovolaemic phase – patient with pallor, sweating with a thready pulse.

There are several *diagnostic* criteria when sepsis is encountered and these are shown in Boxes 19.3 and 19.4.

---

**Box 19.3** Criteria 1 when considering if a patient has sepsis

**Known or strongly suspected infection**
**And any two of the following:**
   Fever or hypothermia (temperature >38°C or <36°C)
   Tachycardia: heart rate >100/min
   Tachypnoea: respiratory rate >20/min or spontaneous
      $PaCO_2 < 4.3\,kPa$
   WBC >12 000/mm$^3$ or <4000/mm$^3$
**or a clinical suspicion**

---

**Box 19.4** Criteria 2 indicating hypoperfusion or organ failure

**Any ONE of these:**
   Systolic BP, 90 mmHg or mean arterial pressure (MAP),
      70 mmHg for more than 1 h
   Urine output, 0.5 ml/kg/h for more than 1 h
   Deteriorating level of consciousness (not due to sedation or
      known CNS disease)
   Metabolic acidosis: pH, 7.30 + base deficit. 5 mmol/l or
      lactate. 4.0 mmol/l

---

If criteria 1 and 2 are fulfilled the diagnosis of Sepsis Syndrome or severe sepsis is made. The time of diagnosis should be documented. This is a medical emergency and the patient's consultant should be informed. The following ward and HDU actions should be taken in the *first hour*:

• 100% oxygen via a rebreathing oxygen mask
• Early fluid resuscitation (as much as 20 ml/kg immediately)

- Blood cultures (as well as genital tract, sputum, urine and line swabs)
- Broad spectrum antibiotics prescribed (with microbiologist advice)
- Broad spectrum antibiotics *given*
- All blood specimens taken including CRP
- Urinary catheterisation
- Lactate sample taken
- Check whether all these steps have been done after 1 h.

It is important to plan for ongoing care of the patient. Identify the source and ensure that continuous antibiotics are being given. Take cultures before giving antibiotics and swab all likely sites. It is important to remember that 75% of cultures are positive from the primary source and about 20% of blood cultures are positive in severe infections.

## Investigations

These are summarised in Box 19.5.

---

**Box 19.5**  Investigations in sepsis

*FBC* – WBCs up or down, platelets normal or down
*CRP* – elevated with a rising trend
*Coagulation screen* – disseminated intravascular coagulation
*Urea and electrolytes* – renal impairment
*LFTs* – liver dysfunction, hypoalbuminaemia
*Electrocardiograph* – dysrhythmias or ischaemia
*Blood gases* – hypoxaemia, acidosis
*Blood cultures* – aerobic and anaerobic
*Other cultures* – high vaginal, sputum, urine, drains, wound, catheters
*Specific* – chest X-ray, ultrasound, CT scan, laparotomy

---

## Management

Immediate management of the patient must be followed by ongoing 6 hourly management plans. Appropriate broad spectrum antibiotics are used initially after consultation with a microbiologist. This is summarised in Box 19.6.

**Box 19.6** Acute management plan for septic patient

Oxygen – up to 100%
IV fluid resuscitation
Monitoring – clinical and technical
Recording – HDU chart noting trends
Physiotherapy
Drugs
   DVT prevention
   Therapeutic antibiotics
   Co-morbid conditions
Management of concomitant obstetric conditions

## Antibiotic resistance

An ongoing unstable patient or a patient failing to progress is a source of great concern. Alerting features include ongoing pyrexia, tachycardia, tachypnoea and rising trends in white cells, CRP and an acidosis mean that a microbiological review must occur. The antibiotics whilst seemingly appropriate may need changing because of bacterial resistance. Of special importance are the extended-spectrum-beta-lactamase enzymes which are now prevalent in bacteria and produce antibiotic resistance. These enzymes now exist in both the community and hospital population. A newer enzyme (CTX-M) produced by *E. coli* is becoming prevalent, and bacterial resistance is becoming more common. This is becoming a challenge and infectious diseases' consultants, physicians and microbiologists must be involved in the discussion of the choice of suitable or additional antibiotics.

If in the first 6 h after diagnosis the patient is still hypoperfused despite fluid therapy and a normal CVP measurement, i.e. hypotensive, oliguric (<30 ml/kg/h) or a serum lactate >4 mmol/l, ITU care must be sought. The patient may need inotropic support, ventilation, appropriate DVT prevention, stress ulceration prophylaxis, insulin therapy and steroid therapy and this care is provided within the ITU.

## Necrotising fasciitis

This is a rare, potentially fatal, condition mainly caused by mixed aerobes and anaerobes. Severe systemic sepsis quickly evolves in conjunction with a haemorrhagic bullous spreading rash. There is underlying fascial and muscle oedema, necrosis and gangrene. The diagnosis is *clinical* and early surgical debridement is necessary. Once the diagnosis is suspected further investigations, e.g. CT scanning for tissue oedema and air, should not delay surgical debridement. In all septic patients this diagnosis must remain within the differential diagnosis.

# CHAPTER 20

# Abdominal pain and jaundice

## Abdominal pain

Wisdom dictates that an early diagnosis leads to the best prognosis, but the differential diagnosis of abdominal pain in pregnancy is a huge challenge. Seemingly well women can mask serious intra-abdominal pathology. Occasionally, dual pathology exists. The ill patient with obstetric complications can have a second pathological process.

The causes can be divided into two groups:
- Obstetric
- Non-obstetric

### Obstetric

The differential diagnosis is 'as long as an arm' and to distinguish the causes are not easy. The important causes that need exclusion are referred to in Box 20.1. A surgical opinion is always useful.

---

**Box 20.1** Obstetric causes of abdominal pain

Severe pre-eclampsia/HELLP syndrome
Acute polyhydramnios
Abruption placenta
Urinary retention
Labour
Uterine fibroids
Acute fatty liver of pregnancy (AFLP)

---

*Handbook of Obstetric High Dependency Care*, 1st edition. By © D. Vaughan, N. Robinson, N. Lucas and S. Arulkumaran. Published 2010 by Blackwell Publishing Ltd

In severe pre-eclampsia or in the HELLP syndrome an early diagnostic sign of disease severity can be abdominal pain. The pain is typically epigastric and right hypochondrial and may be associated with nausea and vomiting. Blood tests as shown below are indicated, and an abdominal ultrasound may be needed to exclude a sub-capsular hepatic haematoma. This must be excluded due to the risk of rupture. Acute polyhydramnios cause sudden and rapid abdominal distension with generalised abdominal pain. The uterus is tender and tense and an ultrasound examination is mandatory. Simple causes such as urinary retention need exclusion in non-specific causes. Acute onset of abdominal pain from 'red degeneration' of a uterine fibroid is not uncommon and complicates term pregnancies.

**Non-obstetric**

The non-obstetric causes are shown in Box 20.2.

---

**Box 20.2**  Common non-obstetric causes of abdominal pain

Acute appendicitis

Gastric ulcer with or without perforation – often not drug (NSAID) related

Infections – acute pyelonephritis, cholecystitis, pneumonia

Urinary calculi

Rupture of liver, spleen and aneurysms (traumatic, cysts congenital abnormalities)

Pancreatitis

Metabolic – diabetic ketoacidosis

Constipation

Domestic violence

---

Delay in diagnosis and treatment of *appendicitis* can lead to maternal and fetal death. The diagnosis is more difficult because the early symptoms of mild pain, anorexia, nausea and vomiting are not unusual in normal pregnancy. Abdominal pain is a consistent finding but the location of the pain may vary and is not uncommonly in the right hypochondrium. Guarding and abdominal rigidity may be lessened. Pyuria may occur which means that a mistaken diagnosis of acute pyelonephritis can be given to the patient.

In *acute pyelonephritis* there is often flank pain and chills or rigours. The patients are pyrexial whereas in appendicitis the patient may be apyrexial. In pyelonephritis there is costo-vertebral tenderness, and urinalysis reveals bacteriuria and pyuria. Urine culture and sensitivity is mandatory. Drugs such as NSAIDs cause gastric perforation and an acute peritonism. *Urinary calculi* cause sharp, severe flank pain, haematuria, frequency and dysuria. Nearly all cases of acute cholecystitis are caused by gall stones at term. Pain in the right hypochondrium is suggestive of this rare disease. Ultrasound diagnosis often helps differentiate the diagnosis of these serious causes.

## Investigations

The necessary investigations for the patient with abdominal pain are shown in Box 20.3.

---

**Box 20.3** Abdominal pain investigations

Full blood count
Urea and electrolytes
Liver function tests
Serum amylase
Urinalysis and culture
Blood cultures
Chest X-ray
Ultrasound
MRI scan

---

The white cell count is indicative of infection or inflammation. A normal white cell count may occur in appendicitis. Vomiting may cause dehydration and hypokalaemia. The liver function tests will reveal a hepatic cause. An erect chest X-ray will show 'gas under the diaphragm' if perforation has occurred. Ultrasound and an MRI scan will assist with the diagnosis of stones (both renal and gall) and may assist in the diagnosis of infections, but a negative scan does not exclude the diagnosis.

## Management

The patient with acute abdominal pain needs care as with any ill patient based on the guidelines shown in Box 20.4.

---

**Box 20.4** Guidelines for treatment of the patient with abdominal pain

History
Examination
Oxygen therapy
IV fluids
Monitoring devices in place
Analgesia
Investigations
Aetiology
   Obstetric?
   Non-obstetric?
   Dual pathology?
Surgical/gastroenterology opinion
Conservative treatment
Surgical treatment

---

## Vomiting

This with nausea are non-specific signs but can be early indicators of severe illness. The differential diagnosis for common causes is shown in Box 20.5.

---

**Box 20.5** Common causes of vomiting

'Physiological' throughout pregnancy
Obstetric causes – pre-eclamptic toxaemia (PET), HELLP, AFLP
Drug induced – opiates, tocolytics
Infections – urinary, gastroenteritis, cholecystitis
Metabolic – hyperglycaemia, uraemia
Surgical – post-operative ileus – nasogastric tube?

---

The cause must be sought and not ignored. The risks of ongoing vomiting relate to hypokalaemia and dehydration. IV fluids with potassium supplementation must be considered depending on the electrolyte results.

## Jaundice

Jaundice is a serious sign, and medical and surgical advice must be sought. The physiological changes of increased liver metabolism in pregnancy mean that interpretation of LFTs is complicated. Simply speaking, serum alanine transaminase (ALT) and aspartate transaminase (AST) decrease by about a third at term. Albumin remains unchanged. Fibrinogen increases and most significantly the alkaline phosphatise rises dramatically from two to four times from non-pregnant levels. Occasionally it is raised up to eight times the normal level in isolation, and this is normally of placental origin.

Causes of jaundice are divided into obstetric and non-obstetric. These causes are listed in Box 20.6.

---

**Box 20.6**  Causes of jaundice

**Obstetric**
  Obstetric cholestasis
  AFLP
  HELLP syndrome

**Non-obstetric**
  Hepatitis A, B, C, D, E
  Herpes simplex virus
  Gall bladder disease

---

Diagnosis is essential. The changing patterns of LFTs in various conditions are discussed in Chapter 25. Treatment is supportive and aimed at preventing liver failure. Acute liver failure is defined as the onset of hepatic encephalopathy within 8 weeks of presentation and in the absence of pre-existing liver disease. It is further sub-defined by the terms 'hyperacute' (encephalopathy within 8 days of jaundice onset), 'acute' (8–28 days) and 'subacute'

(4–26 weeks). Hepatic encephalopathy is clinically classified into four grades:

1 Altered mood: rousable and coherent, impaired intellect, concentration and psychomotor function
2 Inappropriate behaviour: rousable and conversant, increased drowsiness and confusion
3 Stuporous but rousable: often agitated and aggressive
4 Coma: unresponsive to painful stimuli.

The management of the patient with developing acute liver failure is outlined in Box 20.7.

---

**Box 20.7** Management of acute liver failure

Correct diagnosis
Medical/surgical advice sought
Need for ITU considered
Need for transfer to acute liver unit considered
Cardiovascular – hypovolaemia due to vomiting is not uncommon, IV crystalloids need to be given to avoid dehydration
Renal – ARF due to dehydration is not uncommon. Early renal support may be necessary
Haemorrhage – severe coagulopathy possible
Encephalopathy – cerebral oedema means cerebral function needs monitoring
Infection is common
Nutrition status: advice needed, enteral feeding may be needed

# CHAPTER 21

# Management of pain on the MHDU

Provision of high quality pain relief is essential to the management of any obstetric patient. Aside from the humanitarian reasons there are sound medical reasons to ensure good analgesia is provided to all obstetric patients. The risk of thromboembolic disease, which is already increased in pregnancy, may be further exacerbated by immobility, secondary to pain. Reduced mobility can also increase the risk of respiratory complications. Inadequate analgesia may impair a mother's ability to care for and bond with her baby. This includes the initiation of breastfeeding. These issues are of particular importance for a mother who has suffered a complication of pregnancy and childbirth necessitating admission to the MHDU. A further consideration in the MHDU patient is that good analgesia will contribute significantly to ensuring cardiovascular stability, e.g. in the pre-eclamptic/eclamptic patient.

There is very little specific information available about the provision of analgesia to the MHDU patient or indeed the maternity patient in the ICU. Most of the studies on post-operative analgesia in the obstetric patient refer to women who have had elective caesarean sections, usually under regional anaesthesia, and who will have had psychological preparation (information sheets, etc.). Furthermore the women in these studies would have had relatively 'short term' severe post-operative pain. Women admitted to the MHDU may not have had caesarean sections but could still experience significant perineal/peri-anal pain following instrumental delivery and episiotomy. Despite these issues, much of the available information about analgesia will be applicable to the MHDU patient. There are, nevertheless, some important considerations

*Handbook of Obstetric High Dependency Care*, 1st edition. By © D. Vaughan, N. Robinson, N. Lucas and S. Arulkumaran. Published 2010 by Blackwell Publishing Ltd

regarding analgesia in the MHDU patient, which need to borne in mind when providing analgesia (Box 21.1).

Furthermore, the MHDU patient may be antepartum so the effect of any drugs on the fetus must be carefully considered, e.g. NSAIDs should be avoided in the antepartum patient, particularly in the last trimester.

---

**Box 21.1** Important considerations when providing analgesia to the MHDU patient

The MHDU patient:
• May have had an emergency procedure, without adequate psychological preparation
• May have had additional procedures, e.g. hysterectomy
• May require further surgical procedures, e.g. removal of Rusch balloon
• Is more likely to have received general rather than epidural/ spinal anaesthesia
• May be more vulnerable to the side effects of analgesic drugs because of underlying morbidity, e.g. NSAIDs and pre-eclampsia
• Drug absorption/metabolism/excretion may be affected by underlying morbidity
• May be receiving multiple medications – beware of drug interactions

---

## Options for management

As with pain management in all patients, a multimodal approach with regularly administered analgesia is the most effective approach. The NICE caesarean section guideline published in 2004 includes guidance on post-caesarean section analgesia (Box 21.2).

The majority of patients requiring analgesia on the MHDU will have had surgical intervention in theatre prior to admission to the MHDU. Strategies for analgesia begin *before* the patient's admission to the MHDU, while the patient is still in theatre. When a regional technique is used (spinal block or epidural) a dose of diamorphine should be given as per the NICE recommendations.

**Box 21.2** NICE recommendations for post-caesarean section analgesia

- Women should be offered diamorphine (0.3–0.4 mg intrathecally OR 2.5–5.0 mg epidurally) because it reduces the need for supplemental analgesia after caesarean section
- PCA using opioid analgesics should be offered because it improves pain relief
- NSAIDs should be offered to women after post-caesarean section because they reduce the need for opioids, provided there is no contraindication

Women who have a caesarean section should be prescribed and encouraged to take regular analgesia for post-operative pain including:

- For severe pain, co-codamol with added ibuprofen
- For moderate pain, co-codamol
- For mild pain, paracetamol

It may be worth considering leaving an epidural catheter *in situ* to use to provide analgesia on the MHDU either to allow a further dose of diamorphine to be given, or using epidural 'top-ups' with a low dose solution (e.g. bupivacaine 0.1% with fentanyl 2 mcg/ml). However, this will be dependent on local policy and it is essential that there are local protocols available to support such practice. The risk of delayed respiratory depression with epidural opioids should be borne in mind when discharging a patient, who has had repeat doses of epidural opioids, from the MHDU.

In the case of an emergency where the patient received a general anaesthetic but with an epidural catheter *in situ*, diamorphine can be given at the end of the procedure. Similarly if the urgency of the procedure necessitated a general anaesthetic, consideration should be given to surgical local anaesthetic infiltration at the end of the procedure.

In any environment and particularly on the MHDU pain is preferably managed by 'prevention' rather than treatment. Most women are suitable for treatment with paracetamol which when given regularly will have an opioid-sparing effect. Paracetamol is now available as an IV preparation making it particularly suitable for use in the MHDU patient. NSAIDs such as diclofenac may

also be used in the MHDU patient. However, because of their
side risk profile (Box 21.3) and contraindications they may not
be suitable for all women.

---

**Box 21.3** Side effects of NSAIDs

• Gastrointestinal irritation
• Adverse effect on platelet function – prolongation of bleeding
  time
• Aspirin-induced asthma – cross sensitivity with other NSAIDs
• Nephrotoxic – particularly in combination with other
  nephrotoxic agents, e.g. aminoglycoside antibiotics. Caution
  also required in the pre-eclamptic patient

---

Opioids, most commonly morphine, may be given via the oral,
IM and IV route. Patient controlled analgesia (PCA) is widely
used in the non-obstetric population. Analgesia is provided via a
pump which the patient controls and when triggered delivers a set
amount of drug, usually morphine, intravenously. It is significantly
superior to IM opioids and increases patient satisfaction. Despite the
side effects of morphine (respiratory depression, nausea and sedation)
it remains the most popular drug for use with PCAs. Regular anti-
emetics are often prescribed with morphine PCA (e.g. cyclizine
50 mg three times a day) to limit nausea and vomiting. Opioids also
cause constipation, which may already be a problem in the MHDU
patient and consideration should be given to the regular use of laxa-
tives in MHDU patient receiving opioid analgesia. A further concern
is the small but present risk of pressure sores in an immobile patient
with an epidural *in situ*. Although rare, pressure sores have been
described in obstetric patients receiving epidural analgesia.

Most hospitals have a designated acute pain team to maintain
and monitor acute pain management in patients on the wards.
This team is usually made up of a specialist nurse, a pharmacist
and a consultant anaesthetist with a special interest in acute pain
management. The team will review patients on the wards who
are receiving treatment for acute pain usually following surgery.
The maternity unit will not necessarily form part of the acute pain
team's remit, but they can be a useful source of support when
dealing with acute pain management issues on the MHDU.

Lastly, non-pharmacological methods can also contribute significantly to the management of pain in the MHDU patient. Simple measures such as careful positioning of invasive monitoring, urinary catheters, drains, etc. can be helpful. Psychological support is also extremely important. The MHDU patient may be frightened and traumatised by her experience. Kind and compassionate care, while no substitute for good analgesia, can significantly ameliorate the psychological effects of post-operative pain.

A summary of the strategies to manage pain in the MHDU patient is shown in Box 21.4.

---

**Box 21.4** Strategies to manage pain in the MHDU patient

Utilize regional techniques (epidural/spinal anaesthesia) as far as possible. Consider leaving epidural catheter *in situ* if local policy allows.

Consider the use of surgical infiltration with local anaesthetic in those women who have not had an epidural/spinal.

*Regular* analgesia on the MHDU

- Paracetamol or co-codamol
- NSAIDs if no contraindication
- Opioids – oral/IM/PCA

Non-pharmacological methods

- Careful patient positioning
- Psychological support

Advice and assistance from hospital pain team

# CHAPTER 22
# Immobility and thromboembolic disease

The leading cause of direct maternal death in the UK is thrombosis and/or thromboembolic disease and this has been the case for more than 20 years. However, within this group the pattern of disease has changed over the same time period. There has been a decrease in the number of deaths due to pulmonary embolism after caesarean section, almost certainly as a result of increased awareness in the obstetric team and meticulous use of thromboprophylaxis guidelines. This pattern has not been reflected in the number of antepartum deaths where there has been a slight increase since 1985.

The increased risk of thromboembolic disease starts as soon as pregnancy begins. In addition to the physiological changes of pregnancy, the parturient may have pre-existing risk factors. These may be compounded by other factors arising during pregnancy (Box 22.1).

A frank manifestation of thromboembolic disease such as DVT may be the reason for the patient requiring admission to the MHDU, but women admitted to the MHDU for other reasons are likely to have more than one additional risk factor for thromboembolic disease.

Deaths from thromboembolic disease occur mainly because of pulmonary embolism but in consecutive Confidential Enquiry reports there are women who die from cerebral vein thrombosis. There are striking similarities between PE and cerebral vein thrombosis in terms of risk factors.

## Prophylaxis

The gold standard recommendations for thromboprophylaxis in obstetrics comes from two papers from the RCOG – the 'Report of

*Handbook of Obstetric High Dependency Care*, 1st edition. By © D. Vaughan, N. Robinson, N. Lucas and S. Arulkumaran. Published 2010 by Blackwell Publishing Ltd

> **Box 22.1** Risk factors for venous thromboembolism (VTE) during pregnancy
>
> **Pre-existing**
> Previous history of VTE
> Thrombophilia – congenital/acquired
> • Protein S or C deficiency
> • Factor V Leiden
> • Antithrombin deficiency
> • Prothrombin gene variant
> • Antiphospholipid syndrome
> • Lupus anticoagulant
> Age >35 years
> Obesity
> Severe varicose veins
>
> **Factors arising during pregnancy**
> Surgery during pregnancy or puerperium
> Severe infection/sepsis
> Long haul air travel
> Pre-eclampsia
> Massive haemorrhage
> Dehydration
> Prolonged labour
> Immobility

the RCOG Working Party on Prophylaxis Against Thromboembolism in Gynaecology and Obstetrics' and 'Thromboprophylaxis during pregnancy, labour and after vaginal delivery' (Green-Top Guideline number 37) – which are accessible via the RCOG website.

The key area in both documents is assessment of risk factors for thromboembolism in individual patients and risk stratification for subsequent management. Ideally this risk stratification is done as early on in pregnancy as possible, to enable the initiation of thromboprohylaxis if it is required. It is a further recommendation that women should be reassessed before or during labour for risk factors for VTE. It would seem logical to extend this reassessment recommendation to those women who require admission to the MHDU.

A concern highlighted in the 2000–2002 and 2003–2005 Confidential Enquiry reports was the inadequate doses of heparin thromboprophylaxis that women received. It is now well established that heparin requirements for VTE prophylaxis are increased in pregnancy. The RCOG offers guidance on antenatal prophylactic doses of low molecular weight heparin (LMWH), shown in Box 22.2.

---

**Box 22.2** RCOG recommendation for antenatal prophylactic doses of LMWH

|  | **Enoxaparin** | **Dalteparin** | **Tinzaparin** |
|---|---|---|---|
| Normal body weight | 40 mg daily | 5000 units daily | 4500 units daily |
| Body weight < 50 kg | 20 mg daily | 2500 units daily | 3500 units daily |
| Body weight > 90 kg | 40 mg BD | 5000 units BD | 4500 units BD |

---

## Diagnosing DVT on the MHDU

The clinical features of DVT (Box 22.3) are non-specific and making a diagnosis of DVT requires both clinical assessment and objective testing.

---

**Box 22.3** Clinical features of DVT

- Swelling and pain of the affected limb
Physical examination
- Low grade pyrexia
- Tenderness of affected limb
- Increase in circumference of affected limb
- Warmth and redness of affected limb
- Superficial venous dilation
- Positive Homan's test (pain on dorsiflexion of foot)

The RCOG Green-Top Guideline number 28 provides an excellent review of the immediate investigation and management of women in whom VTE is suspected.

The guideline highlights that any woman with signs and symptoms of VTE should be treated with LMWH until the diagnosis is excluded by objective testing (unless treatment with LMWH is strongly contraindicated). It is also highlighted that investigations to confirm or exclude VTE should be performed expeditiously. Compression duplex ultrasound is the most important diagnostic test for DVT. If ultrasound confirms the diagnosis of DVT, treatment with LMWH should be continued. However, if the ultrasound is negative and there is a strong element of clinical suspicion, the woman should continue to receive anticoagulation and the test should be repeated in 1 week. D-dimer testing should not be performed to diagnose DVT in pregnancy because it can often be elevated in normal pregnant women at term and in the puerperium.

## Pulmonary embolism

The end point all these measures are attempting to prevent is a maternal PE, where the clot breaks loose from the leg/pelvic veins and passes through the heart to block the pulmonary arteries and often the right ventricle. The clinical features and relevant investigations are described in Boxes 22.4 and 22.5, respectively.

---

**Box 22.4** Clinical features of pulmonary embolism

PE may be asymptomatic, may present with sudden cardiac arrest, or anywhere in between. The following features reflect increasingly severe disease but may not be found at all:
- Sudden onset pleuritic or central chest pain, worse on exercise
- Haemoptysis
- Variably severe dyspnoea
- Cardiovascular collapse
- Cardiac arrhythmia or arrest

**Box 22.5** Investigation for suspected PE

ECG -- features of severe right heart strain – sinus tachycardia, right axis deviation, right bundle branch block, tall t waves in lead II due to right atrial dilation. The 'classic' $S_1Q_3T_3$ is unreliable at the best of times and is also a normal variant in mid- to late pregnancy
Arterial blood gas – low $PaO_2$ and $PaCO_2$
CXR – usually normal but acutely may show effusion
Definitive diagnosis is radiological, either by *VQ scan* or more commonly a *CT of the pulmonary arteries (CTPA)*

Treatment is initially supportive until the mother is stabilised. Standard therapy is based on LMWH weight-adjusted doses (Box 22.6) though in life-threatening cases thrombolysis, mechanical disruption of the clot with a pulmonary artery catheter and radiological or surgical embolectomy have been used successfully.

**Box 22.6** Therapeutic LMWH doses in PE

Enoxaparin – 1 mg/kg BD
Dalteparin – 90 units/kg BD
Tinzaparin – 90 units/kg BD or 175 units/kg daily

# CHAPTER 23

# Abnormal urine output and renal function

The kidneys are amongst the most sensitive organs of the body. In health no proteinuria or glycosuria occurs but in pregnancy the renal threshold for reabsorption of glucose can be exceeded and proteinuria, of course, is indicative of pre-eclampsia.

The minimally acceptable amount of urine production is 0.5 ml/kg/h. This, in health in an average person, equates to about 25– 50 m l / h or a minimum of 100 ml every 4 h.

Acute renal failure (ARF) is defined as a recent, reversible or potentially reversible deterioration in renal function. It is common with an incidence of up to 7% for hospitalised patients.

## Oliguria

Oliguria occurs when there is less than 0.5 ml/kg/h for one or more hours. A systematic approach to investigation and treatment must occur for the oliguric patient. The causes are categorised into pre-renal, renal and post-renal.

### Pre-renal causes

Pre-renal failure is the inadequate perfusion of otherwise normal kidneys. Renal perfusion requires an adequate blood volume and blood pressure. The pre-renal causes are shown in Box 23.1.

The most important and common causes are hypovolaemia and hypotension.

Abdominal compartment syndrome is intra-abdominal hypertension (>25–30 mmHg) and the relevant causes are faecal peritonitis, retroperitoneal haematoma, intestinal obstruction and post-operative

---

*Handbook of Obstetric High Dependency Care*, 1st edition. By © D. Vaughan, N. Robinson, N. Lucas and S. Arulkumaran. Published 2010 by Blackwell Publishing Ltd

**Box 23.1**  Pre-renal causes of ARF

Hypovolaemia
  Haemorrhage
  Sepsis
  Gastrointestinal losses
  Inadequate intake
Hypotension
  Hypovolaemia
  Cardiac failure
  Vasodilatation
Functional ARF
  NSAIDs
  Hepato-renal syndrome
Abdominal compartment syndrome

complications (particularly haemorrhage). Oliguria, in this syndrome, is caused by reduced total renal blood flow, or from direct renal parenchymal compression. If other causes have been eliminated surgical decompression of the abdomen should be considered. Intra-abdominal pressure is measured from the bladder.

Nephrotoxic drugs are important. NSAIDs inhibit the synthesis of renal prostaglandins which are responsible for afferent renal arteriolar dilatation. In low renal blood flow, NSAIDs may, therefore, cause ARF. ACE inhibitors are also contraindicated in patients such as these. They reduce the production of angiotensin-2 (an efferent arteriolar constrictor which is responsible for maintaining glomerular perfusion pressure). ACE inhibitors are teratogenic. They cause prolonged renal failure in the neonate, decreased skull ossification and renal tubular dysgenesis in the fetus.

The hepato-renal syndrome occurs in chronic renal failure. It is functional renal failure which is characterised by oliguria, high urine osmolality and low urinary sodium. It needs to be distinguished from dehydration and its prognosis relates to the severity of the liver disease.

## Renal causes

Renal causes are due to intrinsic parenchymal renal disease. These are shown in Box 23.2.

---

**Box 23.2**  Renal causes of ARF

Acute tubular necrosis (ATN)
Interstitial nephritis
Glomerulonephritis
Small or large vessel vascular disease

---

ATN accounts for 85% of the intrinsic causes of renal failure. This is a complex disease in which focal damage occurs within the nephron. The proximal tubule cells are vulnerable to hypoxia and undergo apoptosis. Renal biopsy specimens often show little histological damage in this condition. Toxins which cause this condition include inflammatory mediators, aminoglycosides and paracetamol. Renal ischaemia from a reduction in total renal blood flow or the intra-renal redistribution of blood also acts to induce ATN. NSAIDs can further exacerbate the problem by blocking the production of prostaglandin (a renal protector in low flow states).

Interstitial nephritis is caused by an allergic reaction to a drug, an autoimmune disease, infiltrative diseases or infection. Glomerulonephritis is rare and is often related to an intercurrent systemic illness (e.g. systemic lupus erythematosis, SLE). Small or large vessel renal vascular disease can occur and may be thrombotic or embolic.

### Post-renal causes

If both urinary outflow tracts are obstructed ARF will develop. Quick detection and resolution will lead to a complete recovery. The causes are shown in Box 23.3.

---

**Box 23.3**  Post-renal causes of ARF

Intra-renal obstruction from proteins (haemoglobin, myoglobin) or drugs
Renal pelvis (clot)
Ureters (ligation)
Bladder (catheter obstruction)
Urethra (stricture)

---

The most common causes are a blocked or misplaced urinary catheter but the possibility of obstructed, severed or otherwise damaged ureters should be borne in mind.

## Diagnosis and investigations

### History
A careful history and examination normally reveals the likely cause of ARF. Observations will nearly always reveal a period of hypovolaemia or hypotension. The first indication of acutely impaired renal function is oliguria.

### Plasma biochemistry
A rising blood urea and creatinine confirm the diagnosis. A metabolic acidosis occurs with or without hyperkalaemia. Plasma osmolality when considered with urinalysis is also helpful as discussed below.

### Urinalysis
Urinary colour is not a reliable indictor of whether the kidneys are able to concentrate urine. Blood or bilirubin in the urine can cause misinterpretation. It is valuable to note that pre-renal ARF can be distinguished from ATN by urinary and plasma analysis. Urine osmolality, sodium, protein and microscopy help. In pre-renal ARF, the tubules try to restore intravascular volume by reabsorbing salt and water. Sodium concentrations are high in the urine. In intrinsic ARF, the kidneys loose their ability to concentrate and therefore the urinary sodium is low and the urine and plasma are iso-isomolar. Pigmented granular casts are seen in ATN and red cell casts in glomerulonephritis. Typical findings are shown in Box 23.4.

---

**Box 23.4** Urine findings in ATN and pre-renal ARF

| Parameter | ATN | Pre-renal ARF |
|---|---|---|
| Urine osmolality (mosm/l) | <350 | >500 |
| Urinary sodium (mosm/l) | >20 | 10–20 |
| Urinary urea (mmol/l) | <150 | >250 |
| Urine:plasma osmolality ratio | <1.1 | >1.5 |
| Urine:plasma urea ratio | <10 | >20 |
| Fractional excretion of sodium | >1% | <1% |

## Ultrasound

This may help if there is outflow obstruction. A dilated urinary system will be seen. Small kidneys indicate a degree of chronic renal disease.

## Renal biopsy

This is rarely necessary. It is only used if an intrinsic cause other than ATN is likely.

# Management of the oliguric patient

The management of the patient continues from the above and is helped from the history and clinical examination (thirst, cold peripheries, dryness, tachycardia, tachypnoea, hypotension being indicators of pre-renal causes). The management is shown in Box 23.5.

---

**Box 23.5** Management of the oliguric patient

History
   Any obvious event or cause?
Examination
   Signs of hypovolaemia or hypotension?
Ask for advice
Stop nephrotoxic drugs
Blood analysis
Urinalysis
Exclude and manage post-renal causes
   Catheter blocked, kinked, obstructed, or not in bladder?
Exclude and manage pre-renal causes
   Maintain oxygen delivery
   Hypovolaemia – consider fluid challenges
   Hypotension – restore blood pressure
Exclude and manage intrinsic renal causes
   Diuretics, dopamine
   Manage on ITU – dialysis and filtration

---

It is easier to solve the problem in a logical fashion. Exclude and manage post- and pre-renal causes firstly. This will solve 99% of the obstetric population problems.

Post-renal causations are normally easy to solve. The urinary catheter can be blocked, kinked or outside the urinary tract. Flush it and ensure it is correctly sited. If it is sited correctly consider whether any surgery could have damaged the ureters.

Pre-renal causes are often responsible for ARF. The circulating blood volume must be restored. It is acceptable to assess the response to a fluid challenge, e.g. 200 ml boli of colloid or crystalloid can be given incrementally and the response noted. The circulating blood volume can be best assessed from CVP measurements. If hypotension still remains normotension must be restored. This will require advice from an intensivist who may suggest inotropic support for the patient. Noradrenaline or dopamine infusions are used in these circumstances. Adequate oxygen delivery is vital. That means a haemoglobin >8 g/dl and an oxygen saturation > 90% are essential.

Intrinsic renal causes require treatment and any damage is often reversible. Furosemide stimulates the production of vasodilator prostaglandins in the kidney and improves afferent arteriolar nephron blood flow. A bolus dose of 10–20 mg followed by an infusion of 1–10 mg/h may restore an adequate urinary output. Occasionally these measures are inadequate and the patient will require renal replacement therapy (RRT) in an ITU. The indications for this are shown in Box 23.6.

Should any of these parameters be present the patient is normally supported by continuous RRT. Methods used include continuous veno-venous haemofiltration (CVVH) or continuous veno-venous haemodialysis (CVVHD) or haemodiafiltration (CVVDF). These techniques require venous access with a single, wide bore, double

---

**Box 23.6** Indications for renal replacement therapy (RRT)

Fluid overload
Hyperkalaemia (>6.0 mmol/l)
Creatinine rising >100 μmol/day
Creatinine >300–600 μmol/l
Urea rising >16–20 mmol/l
Metabolic acidosis (pH < 7.2)
Clearance of dialyzable nephrotoxins and other drugs
Encephalopathy

iumen cannula. A pump delivers the blood to a filter and the blood is returned to the patient.

If oliguria is from ATN, it is important to remember that the oliguric or anuric phase of ARF lasts typically for 2–4 weeks before a diuresis occurs.

## Polyuria

It is not uncommon for patients in HDU to exhibit polyuria in excess of 200 ml/h for several hours after delivery. However, whilst this may be part of the physiological response to delivery, excessive diuresis has many causes and these are listed in Box 23.7.

---

**Box 23.7** Causes of polyuria

Physiological response to delivery especially in patients with pre-eclampsia
Diabetes mellitus
Diabetes insipidus (cranial or nephrogenic)
Drugs: diuretic therapy
Diuretic phase of ATN

---

Treatment should be observational and supportive in the main with strict attention to the electrolytic state of the patient. Hypokalaemia may develop, and supplementation of potassium may be necessary.

# CHAPTER 24

# Fluid therapy

What fluid should a mother be given for maintenance and replacement of loss? There are three basic forms of fluid replacement therapy that need to be considered when approaching this issue: crystalloids, colloids and blood. Blood transfusion is considered with haemorrhage in Chapter 17.

## Physiology

Total body water (TBW) represents about 65% of the body weight of a term pregnant woman. In a 70 kg parturient about 45 l are water and this is distributed as 66% intracellular fluid (30 l) and 33% (15 l) extracellular. The extracellular fluid is further divided: approximately 12 l as interstitial fluid and 4 l as plasma. Daily requirements include 2–3 l of water, 1–3 mmols/kg of sodium and 1 mmol/kg of potassium.

## Crystalloids

Crystalloids are solutions of ionic or non-ionic particles dissolved in water. There are three commonly used solutions, and 5% dextrose (water) will be considered here as well. Basically the sodium content of the solution determines where these fluids distribute. Higher sodium content solutions (e.g. normal saline) are distributed throughout the extracellular fluid only and lower sodium concentrated solutions (e.g. 5% dextrose) are distributed rapidly throughout the intra- and extracellular fluid compartments. Dextrose saline is a compromise and some people administer this as a routine. Occasionally patients become hyponatraemic if given litres and litres of this solution. This may have serious consequences as

*Handbook of Obstetric High Dependency Care*, 1st edition. By © D. Vaughan, N. Robinson, N. Lucas and S. Arulkumaran. Published 2010 by Blackwell Publishing Ltd

confusion and convulsions can occur. Hartmann's solution most closely resembles extracellular fluid and for this reason is often used in the theatre environment (Box 24.1).

---

**Box 24.1** Composition of commonly prescribed crystalloids and colloids

| Crystalloid | Osmolality (mosmol/kg) | pH | Electrolytes in mmol/l | | | | |
|---|---|---|---|---|---|---|---|
| | | | Na | K | HCO$_3$ | Cl | Ca |
| 0.9% Saline | 308 | 5.0 | 154 | 0 | 0 | 154 | 0 |
| Hartmann's solution | 280 | 6.5 | 131 | 5.0 | 29 | 111 | 2 |
| 4% Dextrose in saline | 286 | 4.5 | 31 | 0 | 0 | 31 | 0 |
| 5% Dextrose | 278 | 4.5 | 0 | 0 | 0 | 0 | 0 |

---

In essence, both 0.9% saline and Hartmann's solution expand the extracellular fluid space and are ideally suited to replace loss from this space. Most clinicians will use either of these two solutions for replacing fluid loss and for maintenance fluids in the delivery suite. Hartmann's solution is probably the best crystalloid to use.

Maintenance of an average mother's intake of 2–3 l/day is essential. In the HDU setting, needs must be balanced by losses (urine, faeces, ongoing from drains). If intravascular fluid expansion is required, normal saline is probably the best solution but excessive usage leads to a hyperchloraemic acidosis.

5% dextrose solution is essentially just water and is not used as a maintenance fluid. It is used as a weak sugar solution for diabetics receiving insulin in the HDU setting and really has no other use.

## Colloids

Gelatins (Haemaccel and Gelofusine) comprise of modified bovine collagens which are suspended in ionic solutions They have long shelf lives and contain molecules of widely varying molecular weight with an average of 35 kDa (for comparison, albumin is 69 kDa). Most of the molecules are small and can be rapidly excreted via the kidneys but they maintain the intravascular volume for some 1.5 h. Only 15% remains in the circulation after 24 h. Anaphylaxis is a rare complication of their usage. Haemaccel contains potassium and calcium.

Hydroxethyl starch is taken up by the reticuloendothelial system after phagocytosis in the blood and this results in its prolonged degradation and elimination. The maximum dose is limited to 20 ml/kg/day. The composition and properties of colloid are shown in Box 24.2.

---

**Box 24.2** Composition (mmol/l) and properties of colloid solutions

| Solution | MW | Plasma $t_{1/2}$ | Elimination | Na | K | Ca | Cl |
|---|---|---|---|---|---|---|---|
| Gelofusine | 30 000 | 3 h | Rapid | 154 | – | – | 125 |
| Haemaccel | 35 000 | 3 h | Rapid | 145 | 5 | 6 | 145 |
| Hydroxethyl starch | 450 000 | 6–9 h | Slow | 154 | – | – | 154 |

---

Colloids are, therefore, ideally suited to replace plasma/blood losses but can be excreted quite quickly and this must be remembered when there is an ongoing situation of fluid loss or haemorrhage.

In summary, as long as the patient has relatively normal kidney function, solutions such as Hartmann's solution are suitable as maintenance fluids. If there is mild haemorrhage or sudden fluid loss (as in severe diarrhoea) colloids are best used to replace and maintain the blood volume.

# CHAPTER 25

# Abnormal blood results

All clinicians in the HDU are confronted by abnormal blood tests and a logical understanding and response needs to be formulated.

## Cell abnormalities

### Normal physiology
There are physiological changes leading to a proportionally greater expansion of plasma volume than the (increased) red cell mass which results in a fall in haemoglobin concentration, haematocrit and red cell count. There is no change in mean corpuscular volume (MCV) or mean corpuscular haemoglobin concentration. The platelet count falls progressively in pregnancy, but should stay within non-pregnant levels. However, levels of platelets can be as low as $100 \times 10^9/l$ in healthy women and thrombocytopenia in pregnancy is considered when the levels are lower than this. The white cell count remains within normal levels in pregnancy.

### Haemoglobin
Anaemia should be suspected when haemoglobin levels are below 10.5 g/dl. In the HDU, anaemia is either pre-existing as a result of normal physiological changes or it arises acutely from haemorrhage. Is the haemorrhage ongoing? If so transfuse if the haemoglobin falls below 8 g/dl. If it has stopped and the patient is stable, consideration to observation and supplementary iron can be undertaken.

### White blood cells
Levels between 4000/mm³ and 12 000/mm³ are normal. Outside of these parameters serious sepsis should be considered and actively

*Handbook of Obstetric High Dependency Care*, 1st edition. By © D. Vaughan, N. Robinson, N. Lucas and S. Arulkumaran. Published 2010 by Blackwell Publishing Ltd

searched for via a septic screen and clinical examination, leading to targeted radiological investigation if indicated.

## Platelets

Elevation of platelets (thrombocythaemia) is rare and is associated with infection, inflammation and the acute phase response after surgery. It is associated with both embolus and haemorrhage. A high count therefore needs treatment. Aspirin 75 mg orally is often used. Low platelet levels (thrombocytopenia) are more complicated. The causes are listed in Box 25.1.

---

**Box 25.1** Causes of thrombocytopenia

Laboratory error – clumping or Coulter counter misread
Gestational thrombocytopenia
Immune thrombocytopenic purpura (ITP)
HELLP syndrome
DIC
Haemolytic uraemic syndrome
Thrombotic thrombocytopenic purpura
HIV infection
Drugs
Sepsis
SLE
Antiphospholipid syndrome
Bone marrow suppression

---

The risks of haemorrhage especially in the mother are real and the cause must be urgently investigated and treated. Haematological advice should be sought early. Platelet packs may be used to replace deficit and caesarean section should only be performed when levels are about 80 000/mm$^3$ unless it is a category 1 section. Corticosteroids are used to stimulate production of platelets in the chronic conditions.

## Coagulation studies

Pregnant women are hypercoagulable but the routine tests of the intrinsic and extrinsic arms of the coagulation pathway (Prothrombin

Time, PT, and activated partial thromboplastin time, APTT) remain normal in health. Anticoagulant therapy minimally raises the APTT. The main worry with coagulation studies is to assess whether the patient is developing DIC. This occurs in the following:
- Haemorrhage
- Pre-eclampsia
- HELLP syndrome
- Amniotic fluid embolism
- Infection
- Fetal death

The diagnosis is made by confirmation of the following: elevated fibrin degradation products (FDPs) and soluble fibrin complexes, lowered fibrinogen and platelets, and prolongation of clotting times. Treatment involves diagnosing the cause and treating the coagulopathy with fresh frozen plasma (FFP), red cells, platelet concentrates and cryoprecipitate.

## Electrolyte disorders

Electrolyte balance can easily become abnormal in the acutely ill mother and every effort should be taken to ensure normality. The major abnormalities will be discussed here.

### Potassium

Potassium is the major intracellular cation. A 70-kg mother has 3500 mmol of potassium of which 60 mmol (2%) is extracellular. The normal range is 3.5–5.1 mmol/l. It is obvious that a large change in total body potassium can result in significant changes in plasma potassium. The daily requirement is 1 mmol/kg in health.

*Hypokalaemia* (<3.5 mmol/l), if mild, is well tolerated. The main causes are shown in Box 25.2.

---

**Box 25.2** The main causes of hypokalaemia

Gastrointestinal losses – hyperemesis, vomiting, diarrhoea
Renal – drugs such as thiazides, loop diuretics, steroids
  – diuretic phase of ARF
  – hypomagnesaemia
  – metabolic alkalosis
Endocrine – hyperaldosteronism, Cushing's syndrome

---

The patient is asymptomatic if the hypokalaemia is mild but if severe cardiac dysrhythmias (tachycardia, SVT and ventricular ectopics) develop and hypertension secondary to sodium retention can occur. The patients can complain of muscle weakness and lethargy, and can develop ileus, cramps, polyuria and constipation. There will be a loss of tendon reflexes in severe cases. The ECG shows a large U wave and flat or inverted T waves. Treatment is by the administration of KCl intravenously at a rate of a maximum of 20–40 mmol/h via an infusion pump.

Hyperkalaemia (>5.5 mmol/l) has many causes and these are shown in Box 25.3.

---

**Box 25.3** Causes of hyperkalaemia

*Factitious* – haemolysed blood sample

*Impaired renal excretion* – ARF, potassium-sparing diuretics, steroid deficiency

*Potassium shift from cells* – acidosis, haemolysis, massive blood transfusion, rhabdomyolysis, post-cardiac arrest

*Other* – iatrogenic (excess intravenously), familial hyperkalaemic periodic paralysis

---

Clinically most patients are asymptomatic until the potassium is >6.0 mmol/l. Confusion and tiredness are associated with the rise. The electrocardiograph shows peaked T waves, flattened P waves and wide QRS complexes.

Management requires exclusion of an erroneous result and then stopping all potassium containing fluids. The treatment options include the following drugs. Intravenous calcium chloride (10%) 10 ml antagonises the cardiotoxic effects of hyperkalaemia and can be repeated immediately. This has an immediate onset and lasts 60 min. It contains 0.68 mmol/ml of calcium. Calcium gluconate 10% can also be used but contains less calcium (0.225 mmol/ml). Bicarbonate 50–100 mmol given intravenously over 20 min has an onset of action of 5 min and lasts up to 2 h. Glucose (50%) 50 ml with 10 units soluble short-acting insulin (e.g. Actrapid) will increase the cellular uptake of potassium. Infusion of beta

2 agonists drives potassium into the cells but there is a risk of dysrhythmia.

## Sodium

Sodium is the main extracellular cation. The normal range is 133–145 mmol/l and the daily requirement is 1–2 mmol/day.

### Hyponatraemia

This is the most common electrolytic disorder seen in the HDU. It is usually associated with an increased body water and is compounded by giving increased hypotonic IV fluids. The causes are listed in Box 25.4.

---

**Box 25.4** Common causes of hyponatraemia

*Water intoxication* – IV 5% dextrose infusion, drugs especially infusions of syntocinon and its derivatives, renal failure
*Oedematous states* – congestive heart failure
Steroid deficiency
*Renal loss* – diuretics, osmotic diuresis (glucose, mannitol)
*Non-renal loss* – vomiting, diarrhoea, peritonitis

---

Clinically symptoms are rare if the sodium is >125 mmol/l but the mother may become confused and have nausea, weakness and cramps. If the level is <120 mmol/l then headache, ataxia, muscle twitching and cerebral oedema (convulsions, coma, respiratory depression) may occur.

Treatment involves firstly following the ABC principles of resuscitation to assessment of the degree of severity of the disorder. Correction of the disorder in the acute phase involves:

- Stopping all hypotonic fluids such as 5% dextrose
- Fluid restriction
- Giving IV frusemide 10 mg boli.

The rate of correction is difficult to dictate as a rapid correction is associated with a morbidity and mortality as a result of the swift decrease in cerebral oedema leading to cerebral osmotic demyelination which leads to permanent neurological damage. For acute symptomatic hyponatraemia the aim is to correct the serum sodium by 2 mmol/l/h until the symptoms resolve (about 20 mmol/day).

## Hypernatraemia

This is rare in the maternity population and results from inadequate urine concentration or losses of hypotonic fluids via the gut. An inability to drink fluids causes the patient to lose their major defence mechanism against hypernatraemia. Administration of water is the priority in treatment.

## Diabetes insipidus

This is caused by impaired reabsorption of water by the kidney. Water reabsorption is regulated by antidiuretic hormone (ADH). The causes are many but in the obstetric population raised intracranial pressure, drugs (phenytoin, ethanol, lithium), chronic renal failure, sickle cell disease and hypokalaemia can all cause it.

## Magnesium

Magnesium is a commonly used drug in the prevention and treatment of eclampsia. It is essential for normal enzyme and cellular function. The total body store is about 1000 mmol of which 60% is in bone. The normal range is 0.7–1.0 mmol/l and the daily input is 10–20 mmol which is balanced by urine and faecal loss. Regulation is controlled by the kidney. Hypomagnesaemia is found in about 65% of critically ill patients and is often associated with hypokalaemia. Magnesium has many general uses including:

• Antacid
• Purgative
• Cardiac dysrhythmias (both ventricular and supraventricular) treatment
• Asthma
• Pre-eclampsia and eclampsia.

In the acute situation it is given intravenously in a dose of 4 g over 5–10 min with an infusion of 1 g/h for 24 h. The side effects of magnesium treatment include warmth, flushing and slurred speech, loss of deep tendon reflexes, and in severe toxicity respiratory depression, respiratory and cardiac arrest with systole.

Treatment of overdose or toxicity includes drug withdrawal and 10 ml IV calcium gluconate 10%.

## Urea and creatinine

Urea elevation is a sign of protein catabolism and this can happen in haemorrhage mainly in the HDU situation. Elevation of creatinine is serious and a sign of renal failure. Early involvement of nephrologists is vital, and baseline investigations include exclusion of post-renal failure due to catheter blockage and renal ultrasound.

## Liver function tests

The physiological changes in pregnancy at term are shown in Box 25.5.

---

**Box 25.5** Physiological changes in LFTs at term compared to non-pregnant levels

*Bilirubin* – lower limits of normal or small reduction
*Total protein* – lowered to two-thirds non-pregnant level
*Albumin* – lowered minimally or normal
*AST, ALT, gamma glutamyl transerase (γGT)* – lowered to two-thirds non-pregnant levels
*Alkaline phosphatase (ALP)* – raised fourfold

---

Liver dysfunction associated with critical illness is common but acute liver disease in itself is a rare cause of admission to the HDU. Cholestatic liver disease is associated with pre-eclampsia. In pre-eclampsia abnormal LFTs can occur as a result of liver congestion or alterations in liver perfusion. Specifically elevated lactate dehydrogenase (LDH), AST and ALT can occur. Abnormal LFTs occur as part of the HELLP syndrome which is associated again with pre-eclampsia.

The patterns of liver function associated with liver disease are shown in Box 25.6.

**Box 25.6** Patterns of liver function associated with liver disease

|  | AST/ALT | γGT | ALP | Bilirubin |
|---|---|---|---|---|
| Cholestasis |  |  |  |  |
| Intrahepatic | ++ | ++ | ++ | +++ |
| Extrahepatic | + | ++++ | ++++ | ++++ |
| Cirrhosis |  |  |  |  |
| Alcoholic | + | ++++ | + | + |
| Primary biliary cirrhosis | + | +++ | ++ | + |
| Hepatitis |  |  |  |  |
| Chronic active | ++ | ++ | + | + |
| Acute viral | ++++ | ++ | + | ++ |
| Drug induced | ++ | ++ | + | ++ |

## Complement reactive protein

Levels are zero or low (0–5 mg/l) normally and rise in inflammatory processes. Elevation and a rising trend mean sepsis until proven otherwise.

# CHAPTER 26
# Anaphylaxis

Anaphylaxis is a severe, life-threatening, generalised or systemic hypersensitivity reaction. It occurs as a response to either drugs or other allergens (e.g. latex, bee stings etc.) and is a medical emergency which needs an instantaneous response. Prompt treatment, with an emphasis on the early use of adrenaline will usually lead to a successful outcome. Rarely anaphylaxis manifests itself as sudden death in a mother but often the symptoms are mild and as there may be other causes of the symptoms the diagnosis can be delayed. Keep the possibility of anaphylaxis in the back of your mind always. Anaphylaxis can occur immediately or for up to an hour after drug or latex exposure.

## Recognition and diagnosis

The signs and symptoms are shown in Box 26.1.

Only one third of patients who have anaphylaxis will have had previous drug exposure. The major cause of anaphylaxis in the obstetric unit is antibiotics and whilst only a minority of patients who report allergy have true allergy, the consequence of anaphylaxis to IV antibiotics may be catastrophic and self-reporting should be taken seriously. Asthmatics and smokers who have had multiple courses of antibiotics are more at risk. Penicillins and cephalosporins are responsible for 70% of antibiotic-induced anaphylaxis. Other causes include NSAIDs, IV colloid administration, heparins, oxytocin and chlorhexidine.

*Handbook of Obstetric High Dependency Care*, 1st edition. By © D. Vaughan, N. Robinson, N. Lucas and S. Arulkumaran. Published 2010 by Blackwell Publishing Ltd

Latex hypersensitivity is an increasing cause of anaphylaxis and is commonly found to present some 30 min after the advent of surgery such as in a caesarean section.

---

**Box 26.1** Signs of severe allergic drug reactions

Pruritis
Flushing
Erythema
Coughing
Nausea, vomiting, diarrhoea
Angioedema
Laryngeal oedema with stridor
Bronchospasm with wheeze
Tachycardia, bradycardia
Hypotension
Cardiovascular collapse
Disseminated intravascular coagulation

---

## Immediate management

This needs to be second nature to the team caring for the patient and is shown in Box 26.2.

---

**Box 26.2** Immediate management of anaphylaxis

Call for help and note the time
If no output, commence cardiopulmonary resuscitation
Remove causative agents (drugs, IV colloids, latex and chlorhexidine)
Left lateral tilt and 100% oxygen
Elevate legs if hypotension
Administer IV adrenaline (0.5 ml bolus of 1:10 000 – several doses may be required)
Administer normal saline or Hartmann's solution (may need up to 10–20 ml/kg immediately)

Sometimes, drugs like adrenaline are presented as concentrations or percentage strengths, but administered in milligrammes or microgrammes rather than a more easily recognised form. To 'translate' . . .

'1 in 1000' = 1 g in 1000 ml and '1 in 10 000' = 1 g in 10 000 ml. So if you are using a 1 in 10 000 solution, the concentration is 1 g in 10 000 ml which is the same as:

1000 mg in 10 000 ml, OR

1 mg in 10 ml, OR

1000 µg in 10 ml, OR

100 µg/ml.

Therefore in anaphylaxis each dose of adrenaline administered is 50 µg.

## Secondary management

The secondary management is shown in Box 26.3.

---

**Box 26.3** Secondary management of anaphylaxis

Administer chlorpheniramine 10 mg intravenously

Administer hydrocortisone 200 mg intravenously

Treat persistent bronchospasm with inhalational or IV salbutamol.
   IV magnesium and aminophylline may also be used

Consider transfer to ITU

Take blood for mast cell tryptase (5–10 ml clotted blood) as
   soon as practical, 2 and 24 h after the episode (liaise with
   the hospital laboratory)

---

The patient must be followed up and referred to a specialist allergy or immunology centre for appropriate testing. She will need to wear a medic-alert bracelet.

## Latex allergy

Anaphylaxis to the latex rubber in surgical gloves may be immediate or delayed for up to 1 h after exposure to latex. Genetically predisposed patients often have life long mild systemic reactions such as itching, swelling, rhinitis, asthma and anaphylaxis. Contact dermatitis can occur in susceptible individuals but the most frequent reaction is an irritant reaction characterised by itching, irritation and blistering at the site of contact.

Several groups are at risk: atopic patients, patients having multiple operations, patients with severe dermatitis on their hands, healthcare professionals, patients with fruit allergies and those with an occupational exposure to latex.

If a patient is latex allergic, avoidance of latex is mandatory. The operating theatre should be prepared the night before to avoid latex particles being released, synthetic gloves used at all times including the preparation of any theatre trolleys, latex-free dressings, drips and tapes must be used. Most departments have a latex-free trolley with appropriate equipment available.

# CHAPTER 27
# Local anaesthetic toxicity

Two local anaesthetic agents are in common use. These are lidocaine and bupivacaine. The choice of drug depends on the speed of onset and the duration of action required. The addition of adrenaline prolongs the duration of action of local anaesthetics but must not be used when there is a risk of injecting it into an end artery as it causes vasoconstriction and thus potential gangrene. The characteristics of these two drugs are shown in Box 27.1.

---

**Box 27.1** Characteristics of local anaesthetic drugs

| Agent | Duration (h) | Maximum dose | |
|---|---|---|---|
| | | Plain (mg/kg) | With adrenaline (mg/ kg) |
| Lidocaine | 1–3 | 3 | 7 |
| Bupivacaine | 1–4 | 2 | 2 |

---

## What does the term % mean?

Local anaesthetic drugs come in vials containing the percentage concentration displayed. The word 'percent' means grams in a 100 ml. From this fact the maximum dose of local anaesthetic to be used can be calculated, e.g. if you are using 1% plain lidocaine in an 80 kg patient:

1% = 1 g in 100 ml which is

1000 mg in 100 ml which simplifies to

10 mg in 1 ml.

---

*Handbook of Obstetric High Dependency Care*, 1st edition. By © D. Vaughan, N. Robinson, N. Lucas and S. Arulkumaran. Published 2010 by Blackwell Publishing Ltd

The maximum dose of lidocaine is 3 mg/kg, so this lady can have a total of 3 × 80 mg = 240 mg and as there are 10 mg/ml she can have a total of 24 ml 1% plain lidocaine. Similar calculations can be made for 2%, 0.5% concentrations.

The maximum dose should not be exceeded when these drugs are used subcutaneously as toxicity will occur. Additionally, giving local anaesthetics accidentally into veins or arteries will also induce anaesthetic toxicity. Toxicity can be mild or severe.

## Signs and symptoms of mild toxicity

The signs of mild toxicity are shown in Box 27.2.

---

**Box 27.2**  Signs of mild local anaesthetic toxicity

Anxiety
Restlessness
Nausea
Tinnitus
Perioral tingling
Tremor
Tachypnoea

---

Mild toxicity requires that the patient be observed in case severe toxicity occurs. Stop administering the drug and observe the patient clinically. It is prudent to observe the CVS and the patient's heart rate and rhythm should be monitored by an electrocardiograph. Mild symptoms normally resolve quickly on drug administration cessation but severe toxicity can develop.

## Signs and symptoms of severe local anaesthetic toxicity

The signs of severe toxicity may occur at the time of injection of the local anaesthetic agent but may also occur for up to 20 min after the drug has been injected. Obstetricians and midwives may inadvertently cause local anaesthetic toxicity when performing procedures relating to specific nerve blocks (pudendal blocks) or when suturing the perineum. Midwives and anaesthetists can cause toxicity from topping up epidural anaesthesia inappropriately. It is important to remember that the cardiac toxic effects of local anaesthetics, especially bupivacaine, are very hard to reverse and prolonged treatment of a patient with local anaesthetic toxicity is needed. The signs and symptoms are shown in Box 27.3.

---

**Box 27.3** Signs of severe local anaesthetic toxicity

Sudden loss of consciousness with or without tonic–clonic convulsions
Cardiovascular collapse
Sinus bradycardia
Conduction blocks
Asystole
Ventricular dysrhythmia

---

## Treatment of severe local anaesthetic toxicity

Intralipid should be stored in the HDU. The immediate management of toxicity is shown in Boxes 27.4 and 27.5.

The safe outcome revolves around a prompt diagnosis and prolonged team treatment of the patient.

---

**Box 27.4** The immediate management of severe local anaesthetic toxicity

Stop injecting the local anaesthetic
Call for help
Maintain airway with 100% oxygen
Anaesthetist may need to intubate trachea to secure the airway
Intravenous access
Control seizures by diazepam bolus 5 mg or magnesium 4 g slowly
Assess cardiovascular status throughout

**Box 27.5** Management of cardiac arrest associated with local anaesthetic injection

Start cardiopulmonary resuscitation as per guidelines
Manage arrhythmias using the same guidelines
Understand that in local anaesthetic toxicity the arrhythmias
   may be refractory to treatment
Prolonged resuscitation may be necessary
   Consider treatment with lipid emulsion
      Bolus intravenous Intralipid 20% 1.5 ml/kg
      Commence infusion Intralipid 20% at 0.25 ml/kg/min
      Repeat bolus injection above twice at 5 min intervals
      After a further 5 min increase infusion rate to 0.5 ml/kg/min
      Continue infusion until stable circulation is restored
Remember cardiac arrest may take 1 h to recover from
If facilities are available cardiopulmonary bypass may be needed
Report case to the NPSA

# Selected bibliography

## Obstetric texts

1. Catherine Nelson-Piercy. Handbook of Obstetric Medicine. 3rd Edition 2006. Informa Healthcare, UK.
2. Thomas F Baskett. Essential Management of Obstetric Emergencies. 4th Edition 2004. Clinical Press Ltd, UK.
3. Arulkumaran S, Symonds IM, Fowlie A. Oxford Handbook of Obstetrics and Gynaecology. 2004. Oxford University Press, UK.

## High dependency and intensive care texts

1. Charles J Hinds, David Watson J. Intensive Care: A Concise Textbook. 3rd Edition 2008. Saunders, UK.
2. Craft TM, Nolan JP, Parr MJA. Key Topics in Intensive Care. 2nd Edition 2004. Taylor and Francis, UK.
3. Andrew D Berstein, Neil Soni. Oh's Intensive Care Manual. 6th Edition 2008. Butterworth Heinemann, Elsevier, UK.
4. Obstetric Anaesthetists Association/Association of Anaesthetists Guidelines for Obstetric Anaesthetic Services. Revised Edition 2005. The Association of Anaesthetists of Great Britain and Ireland, London.

## Nursing texts

1. Mandy Sheppard, Mike Wright. Principles and Practice of High Dependency Nursing. 2nd Edition 2006. Bailliere Tindall, Elsevier, UK.
2. Tina Moore, Philip Woodrow. High Dependency Nursing Care. Observation, Intervention and Support for Level 2 Patients. 2nd Edition 2006. Routledge, UK.

# Index